Tai Chi Chuan

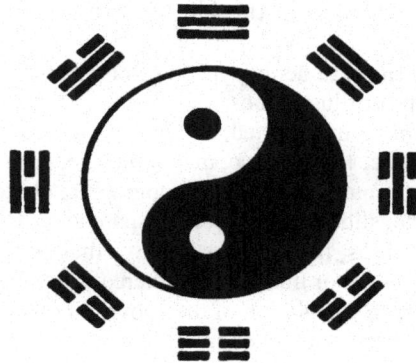

Silk Reeling   Exercises

by

PAUL ELLSWORTH

Tai Chi Chuan, a Moving Meditation for Peace of Mind, Health and
Self Defense

First Edition Published in the United States of America by
Jade Emperor Publishing, P.O. Box 51541, JacksonvilleBeach, Florida 32240-1541.

Photography by James H. Gray

Library of Congress Cataloging-in-Publication Data

Ellsworth, Paul Gerald.
    Tai Chi Chuan Silk Reeling Exercises / by Paul G. Ellsworth
    1. Personal Health and Fitness. 2. Exercises. 3. Tai Chi Chuan. 4. Silk Reeling Exercises (Chan Ssi Ching). 5. Martial Arts. 6. Stress Reduction. 7. Flexibility. 8. Chi Kung Warmups. 9. Chi Development. I. Ellsworth, Paul G. II. Title.

ISBN 0-9710003-1-X
ISBN-13: 9780971000315

The photo on opposite page is the author with student, Joyce C. Morris taken after the book Photo shoot at Memorial Park, Jacksonville, Florida.

For order forms, please see last page.

It is not the intention of the author or publisher to discourage any readers from <u>enjoying</u> these Tai Chi Chuan Silk Reeling Exercises.

Warning - Disclaimer

However, due to the legalities of this society, this disclaimer is necessary. This book presents information and techniques that have been in use throughout the Orient for many years. These practices utilize a natural system within the body. However, there are no claims for effectiveness. The information offered is valid to the author's best knowledge and experience. This information is to be used by the reader(s) at their own discretion and liability. You need to accept legal responsibility for doing a thing you do not thoroughly understand. Because people's lives have different conditions and different stages of growth, no rigid or strict practice can be applied universally. The adoption and application of the material offered in this book is totally your own responsibility.

The author and the publisher of this material are NOT RESPONSIBLE in any manner for any injury, which may occur through reading or following the instructions in this material. The activities, physical and otherwise, described in this material may be too strenuous or dangerous for some people, and the reader (s) should consult a physician before engaging in them.

If you do not wish to accept and be bound by the above stipulations, you may return this book (in an undamaged, like new, resaleable condition) to the publisher for a full refund of the purchase price within three (3) days of purchase. Sales receipt must accompany return.

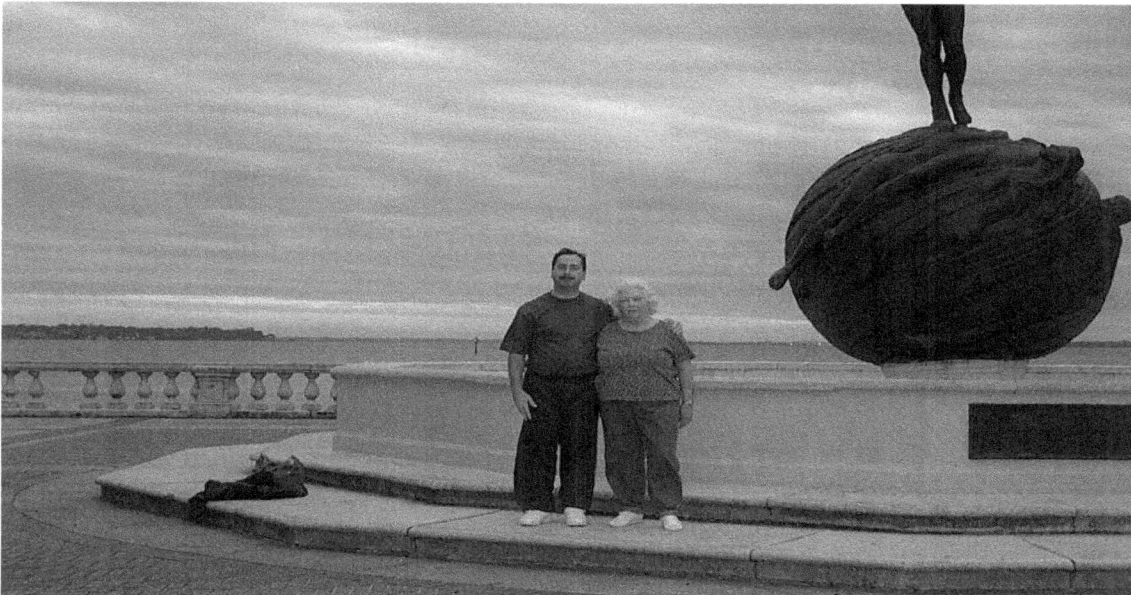

Dedication

To Heaven, thank you for the gift.

To my Mom and Dad, for always being there for me.

To "Sifu", for accepting me as a student;
for making internal real to me;
and for leading me to emptiness.

To those who wish to refine themselves.

To Taoists everywhere past and present.

Acknowledgements

No book is written entirely in isolation. Every author is supported and aided by others. Thanks to my family, sifu (teacher), Kung Fu brothers and sisters, my students, martial arts colleagues and warm personal friends. However, without the help of the following people, this book could not exist:

Gerald P. Ellsworth
James H. Gray
Ken McCray
Joyce C. Morris
Diana Jean Smith
Robert J. Smith

Table of Contents

Preface:
Fundamental Tai Chi Exercises For All Levels

The writing of this book of exercises initially began as a list created by my father. Over a period of time, descriptions and explanations developed and were recorded based on our conversations and training or practice sessions. This was intended to help my dad remember this routine by having reference material when he was practicing on his own.

The primary reason for this was that we did not live in the same town and he traveled on business fairly extensively. Our getting together for review on a regularly scheduled basis was minimal. I have felt (and continue to do so) that martial arts are the perfect traveling exercises available. The specific exercises laid forth in this book can be practiced any place where you can put two feet by anyone with a desire to do them. They can be modified to adjust to the needs of the individual.

The primary purpose of this book is to facilitate the conditioning of oneself through whole body movement. The formal name of these exercises are "chan ssi ching" or "tsan tzi chin" translated from the Chinese language into English as meaning "silk reeling spiraling power exercises". These movements are based upon the concept of the **Circle** and retraining the body-mind-spirit to unify in all things done. It is my highest recommendation for the reader to seek direct training from a properly trained and qualified teacher. This text is intended to be supplemental to live teaching or direct learning experience.

I have been asked over many years by students and friends, "Could you or would you write it down for us?" or "It would be nice if you wrote a book with these exercises in it!". Well, here it is!

It is with my deepest, sincere respect to those teachers (masters) who are familiar with "chan ssi ching" that I ask them to forgive me for my over-simplification to their actual practice. It is not my intention to go into all the deeper internal energy attributes of these exercises in this book. There are higher authorities who can give fuller explanations. It is not the purpose of this writing to go into extensive dissertation on the meditative, philosophical, spiritual or martial application qualities of these exercises. Those may be topics of other books. Yet, I want it understood I feel "silk reeling" is essential to higher levels of Tai Chi for those seeking improved internal development regardless of style.

This series of exercises is my own interpretation of Silk Reeling taught by many masters throughout the generations, specifically as taught by Master F. J. Paolillo. His endorsement is not implied.

I recommend the reader review the written material prior to practicing any of the exercises. Reviewing the Stances is specifically recommended as they are used throughout the routine presented in this book. What is done on one side, should also be done on the other side. If you do 8 counts with your left shoulder, then 8 counts should be done with your right shoulder. If you are physically unable to do an exercise such as a low stance, only go as far as is comfortable until accustomed to the exercise. If you feel pain while doing these exercises,you are most likely doing them incorrectly. This is <u>not</u> a "no pain, no gain" exercise program. Additionally, independent practice of the Stances will improve one's strength and quality of the other exercises. They can also be used as "Chi Kung" meditation postures. Familiarity of the Stances can only improve one's ability.

These exercises were designed to loosen the joints, yet strengthen them such that the internal energy known as "Chi" will circulate freely. To keep this book to the point, I have omitted the discussion of chi development, which will naturally develop through regular practice. "Chan ssi ching" can also be done without having to learn tai chi forms as chi kung development exercises for those who choose to do so. They can stand on their own as they are excellent health exercises.

Paul Ellsworth
Jacksonville Beach, Florida
Year of the Dragon, 2000

You may reach the author by writing to:
Jade Emperor Publishing
P. O. Box 51541, Jacksonville Beach, FL 32240-1541 or send e-mail to:
paul_ellsworth7@yahoo.com

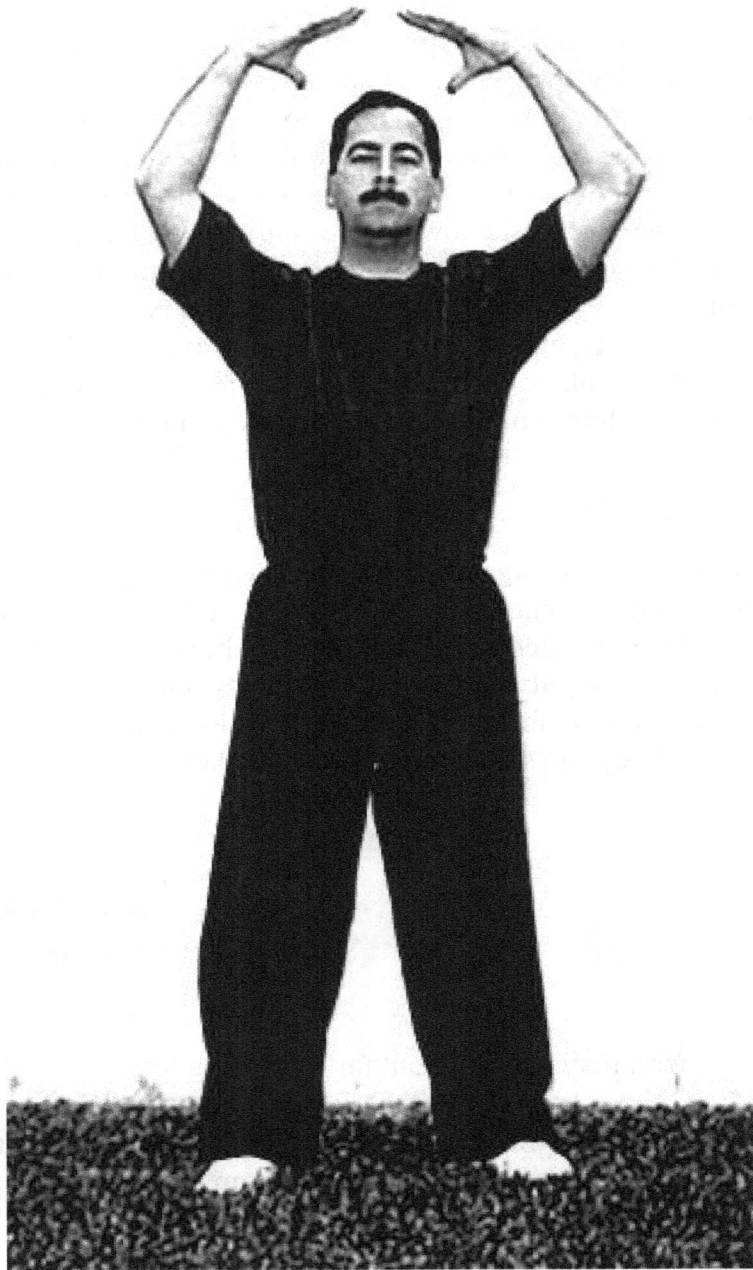

Silk Reeling Routine

1. **Cleansing**: In Neutral Stance, stand upright, knees slightly bent, feet about shoulder-width apart, hands at sides. From lower position, with palms up, inhale through the nose as you raise arms fully extended at side to overhead position; hands covering crown, palms are down, fingers point to each other but do not quite touch. Tongue is up, behind the teeth but not touching teeth. (Like saying the letter "L") Palms down, <u>slowly</u> lower hands in front of body, fingers close but apart. As hands pass in front of upper palate, lower tongue from roof of mouth and exhale through the nose with mouth closed. Exhaling, continue pressing downward with palms until arms are fully extended to lower position with hands settling at sides. Repeat 3 times remembering to breathe through the nose; inhale up, tongue to roof of mouth; exhale down, tongue lowered. (This movement is a preparation of self.) Mentally stay focused on the lower "Tan Tien"*(pronounced don tee-en). **Thereafter, all movement begins first from the Tan Tien, then extends to rest of body through to fingertips, toes, top of head.** (See photos next page.)

*Literally, "Field of Elixir." A spherical area in the body capable of storing and generating Chi. The lower Tan Tien is located a few inches below the navel.

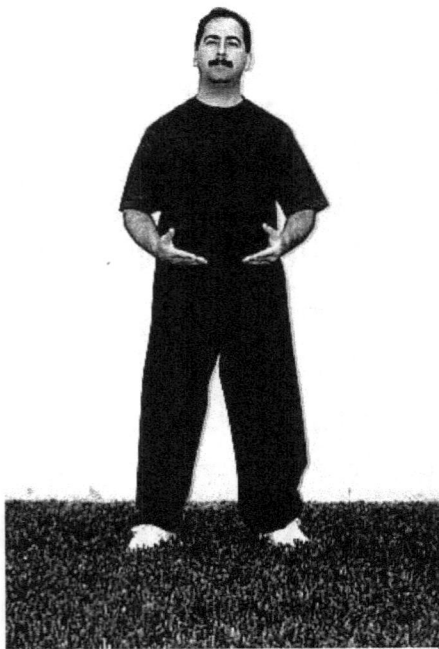 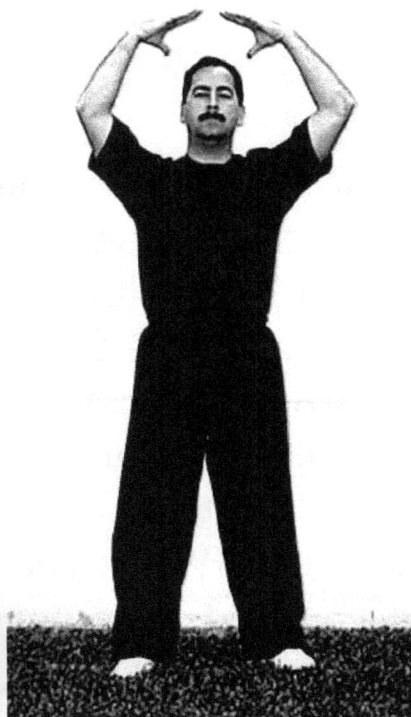 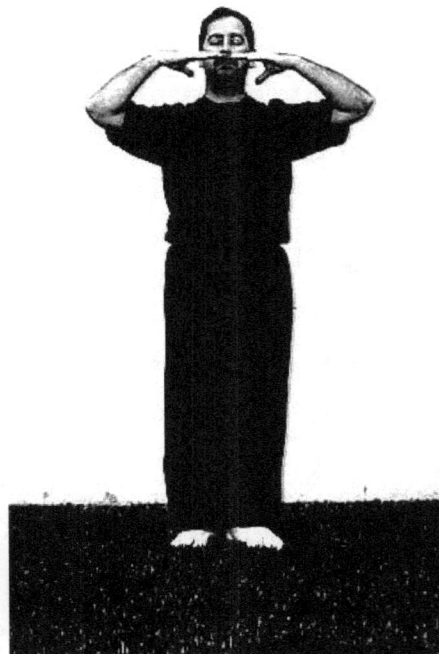

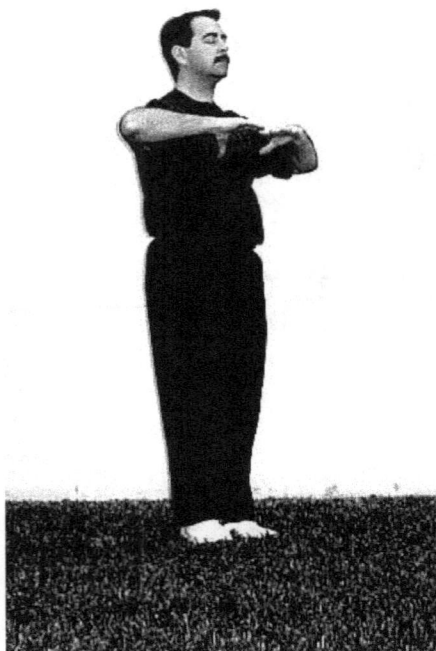 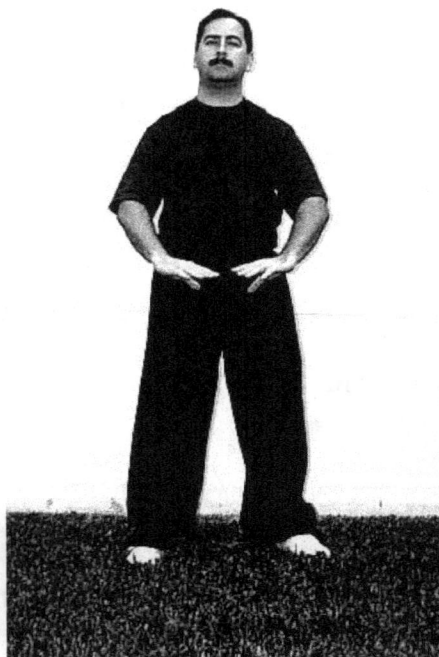 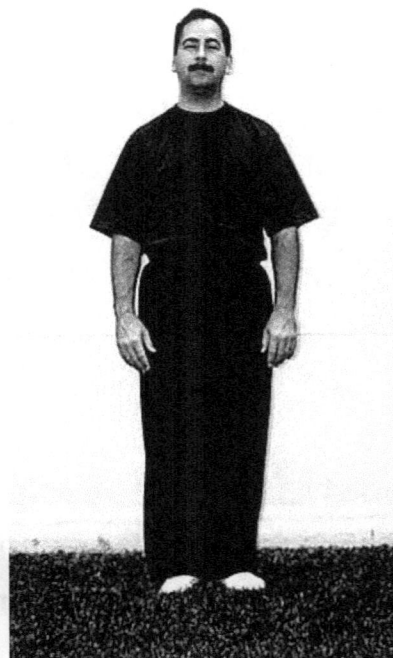

2. **Picking Fruit** - Neutral Stance: Heels together, feet slightly apart; Alternating sides, reach up as though picking fruit from a tree. Always keep a slight bend in elbow instead of letting the elbow lock (i.e. natural extension). Repeat 8 times. Settle - a relaxing pause with arms down at sides.

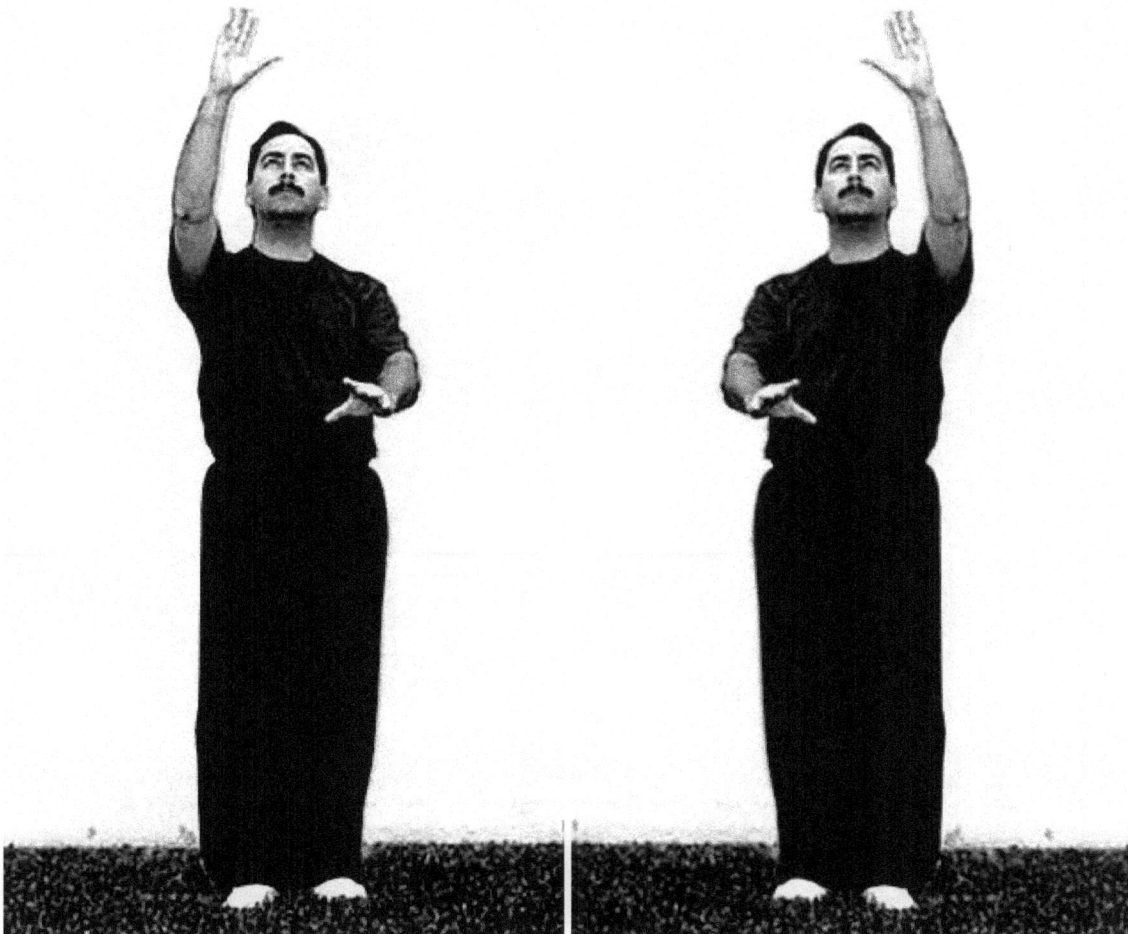

3. **Head** - Left, Right: Neutral Stance, arms down at sides, feet shoulder width apart; Slowly look to left, then right, 4 times; Keep spine aligned, upright; Continuing, move head in left circle 4 times; reverse to right circle 4 times.

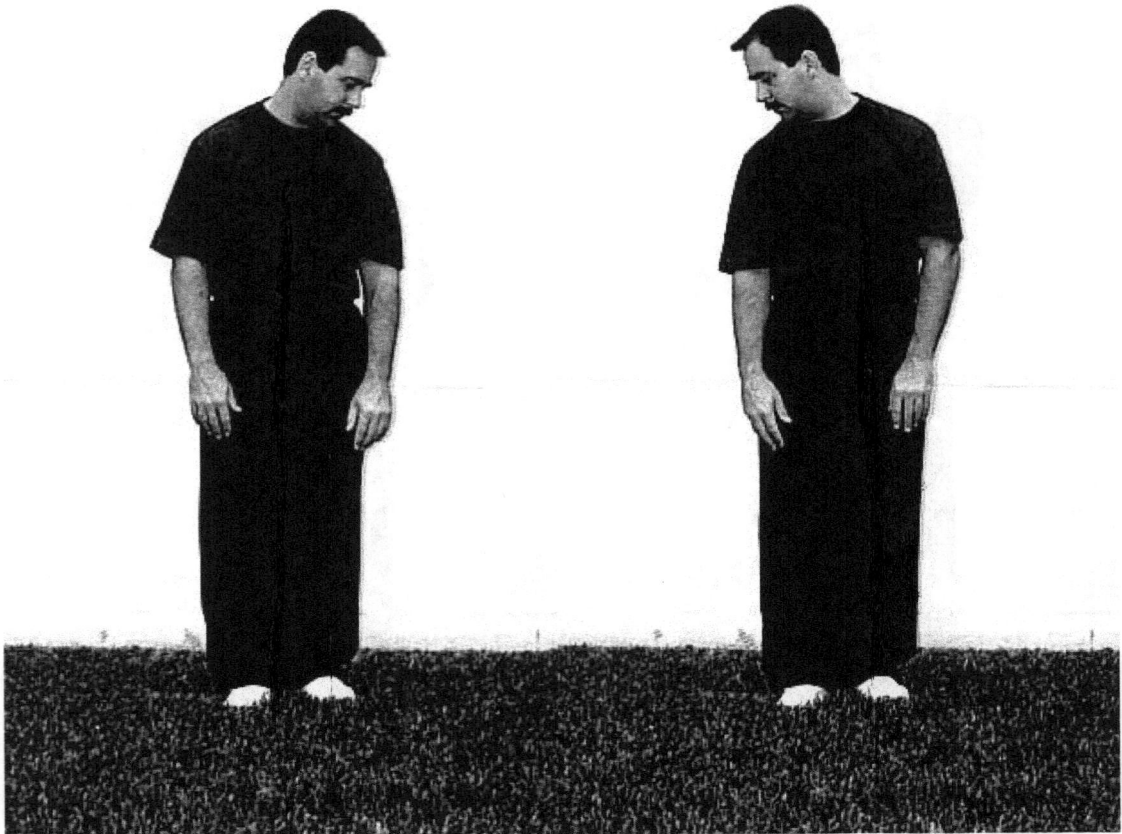

4. **Shoulders** - Left Side, Right Side: Left foot forward, right foot back with toes pointed right, (slightly less than 90 degrees) hands at sides. **As waist turns, from Tan Tien**, left shoulder moves forward, up, back and down in an outside circle (from inside to outside) 8 times. Left hand lightly traces a circle on left thigh. Reverse with figure 8 and lifting shoulder at back, move forward, down, back and up in an inside circle (from outside to inside) 8 times. Reversing feet, repeat the shoulder movement on right side. **(Focus: on use of waist figure 8 motion as origin of shoulder motion.)**

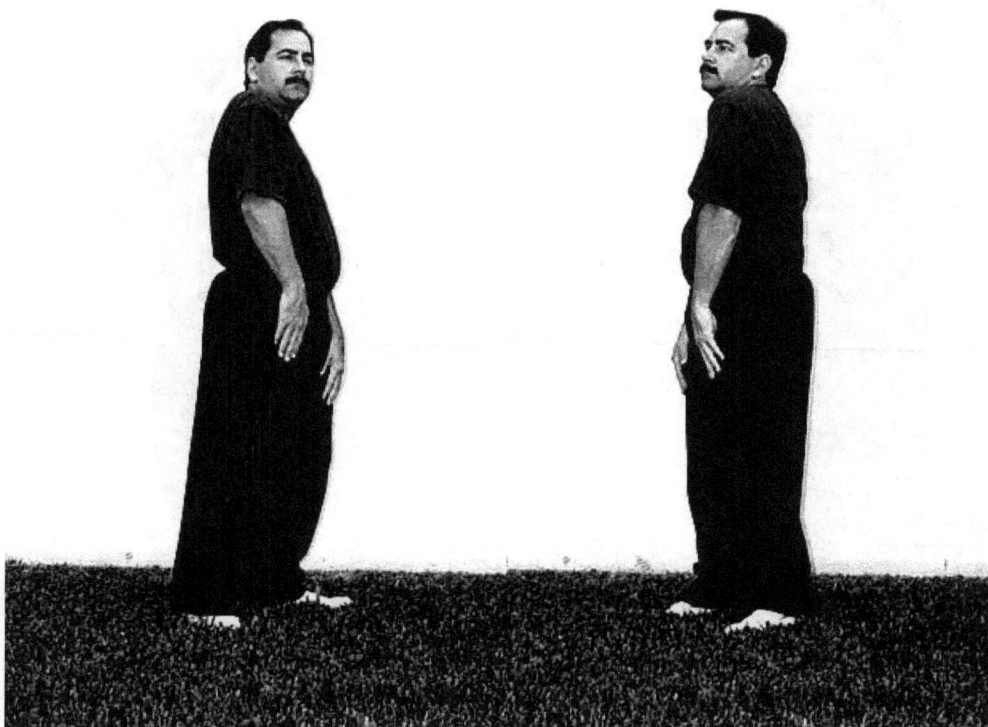

5. **Elbows**: Left foot forward, right foot back as in shoulders, right hand on hip. With left fingers forming a loosely closed fist, lightly touching chest. **As waist turns**, left elbow moves forward, up, back and down in a circle from inside to outside 8 times. Left fist traces a circle on chest. Reverse with figure 8 and, lifting elbow at back, move forward, down, back and up in a circle from outside to inside 8 times. <u>Reversing feet</u>, repeat the elbow movement on right side. **(Focus: on use of hip [waist] figure 8 motion as origin of elbow movement.)**

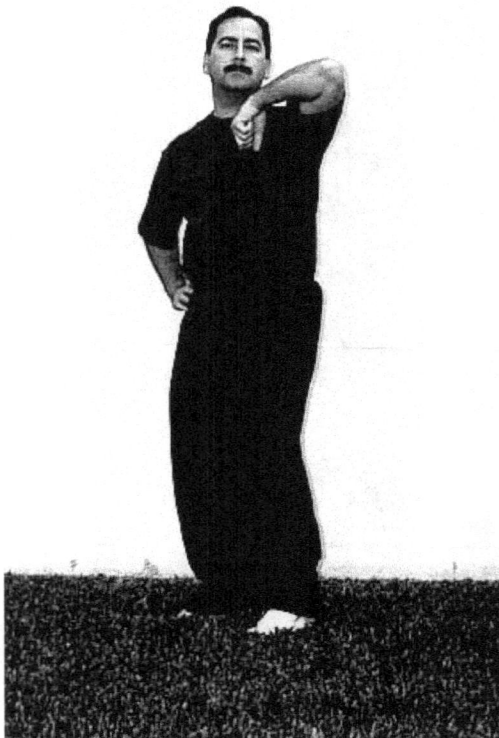

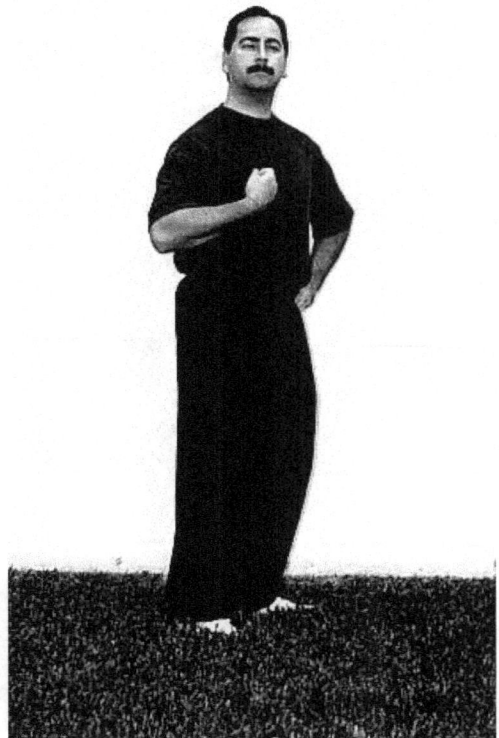

6. **Wrist** - Left Side, Right Side: Left foot forward, right foot back, right hand on hip. Left arm extended, elbow slightly bent. **As waist turns**, wrist turns like a doorknob in a counter clockwise motion 8 times **(outside circle direction).** Reverse direction 8 times **(inside circle direction).** Reversing feet, repeat with right wrist 8 times in each direction.

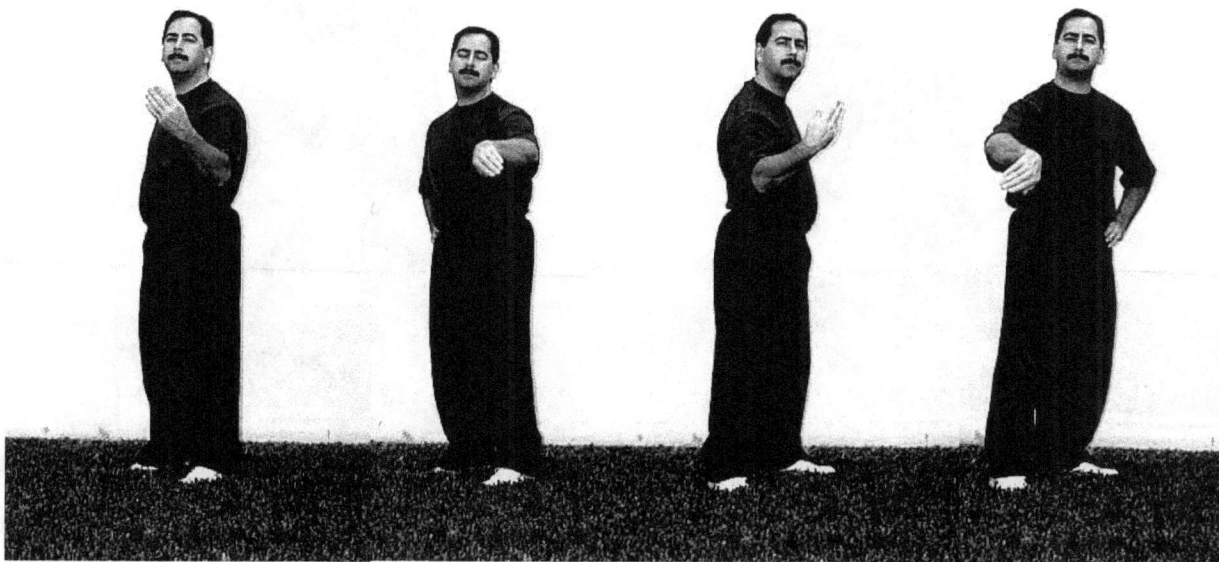

7. **Wrists** - Doubles: Neutral Stance, feet shoulder width apart, extend both arms to the front, elbows not locked. **As waist turns,** move both wrists **inside to outside** 8 times; reverse to move **outside to inside** 8 times.

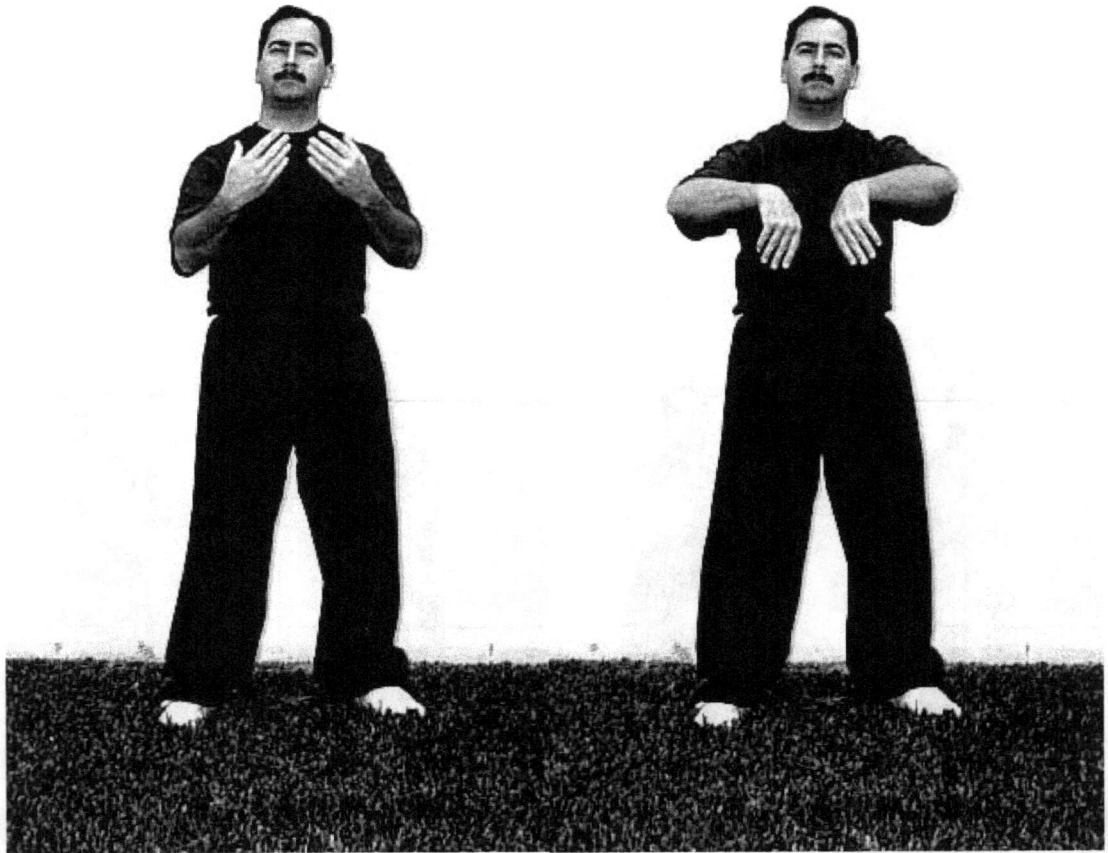

8. **Stir the Chi**: Neutral Stance, with arms extended forward, loosely shake both wrists in front of body.

9. **Cleansing**: (refer to #1 on page 13)

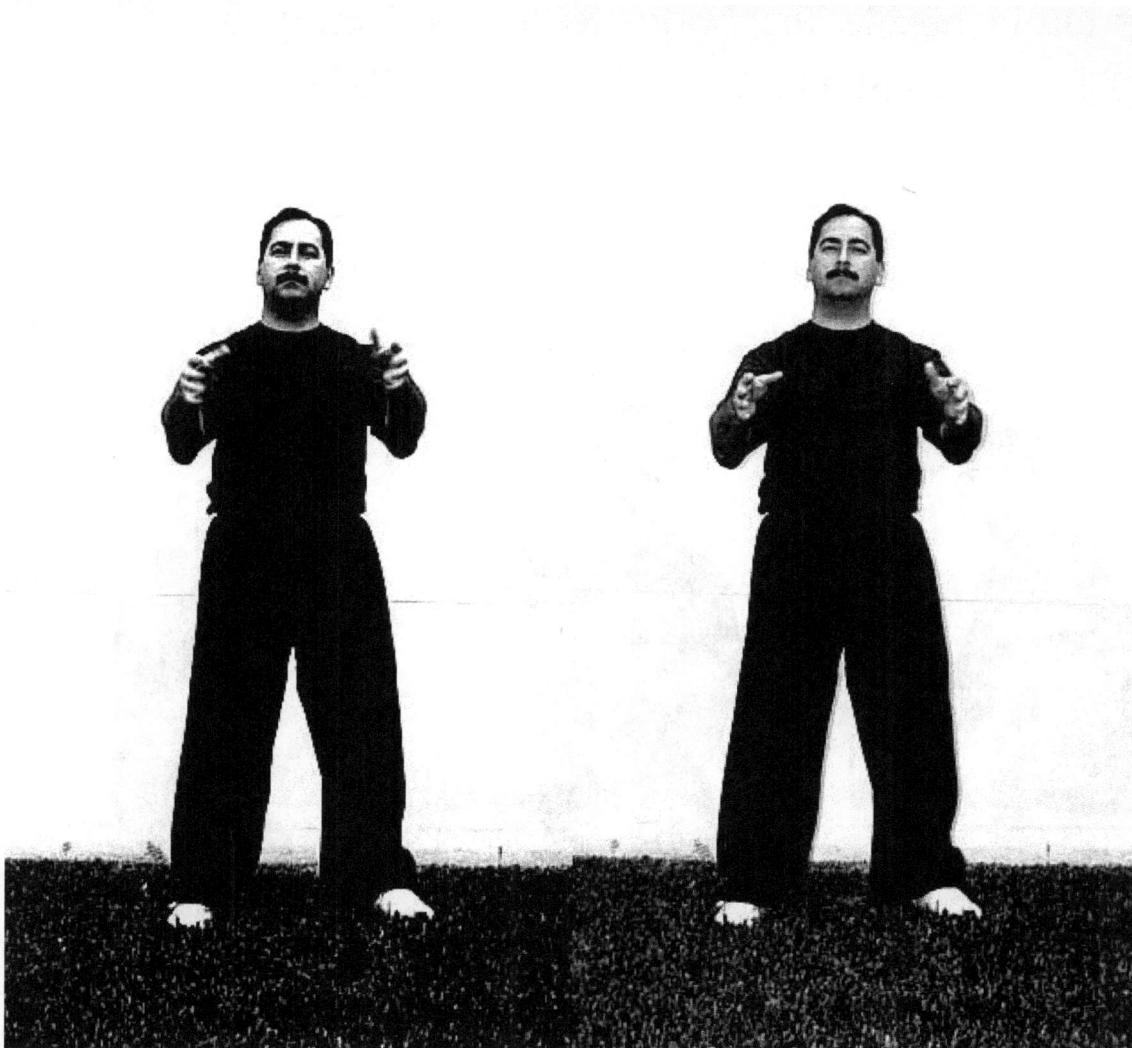

10. **Ward Off** - <u>Left Side, Right Side</u>: Left foot forward, right foot back, right hand on hip; **As waist turns from Tan Tien**, left hand, palm up, moves down, then across body in circle to scoop up water. When fully extended, the arm draws back and out with palm down completing the circle beside the body. Repeat smoothly 8 times. <u>Reverse feet and hands</u> and repeat with right side.

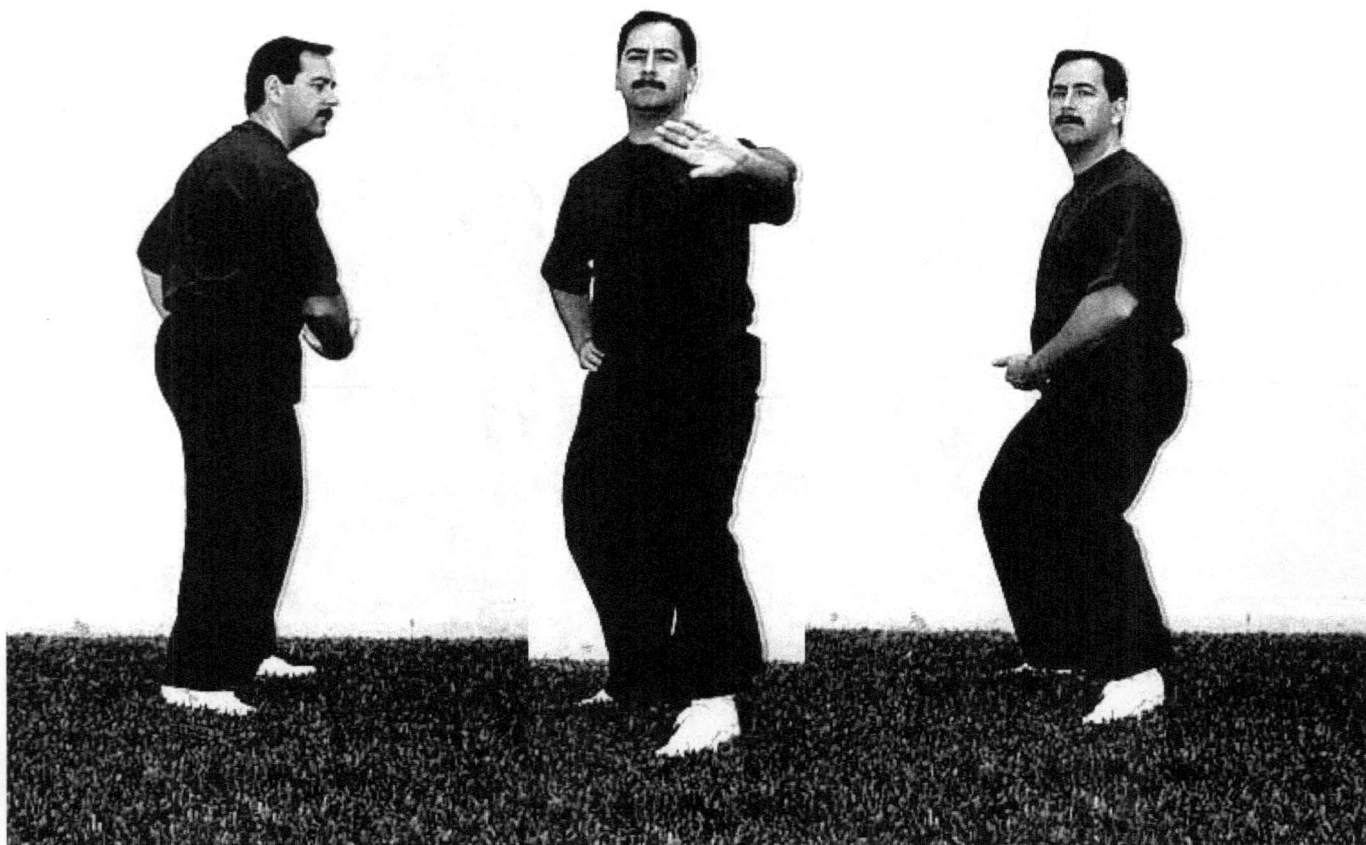

11. **Bend Forward and Back** - Left, Right: Left foot forward, right foot back, hands form loose fist; elbows not locked, arms extended to each side and head up; Using the legs, lean back, then bend forward bringing fists down and back at sides. Reverse by bringing fists up and out to sides while leaning back slightly. Head remains up so eyes can see the horizon throughout forward and backward motion. **Breathe from Tan Tien.** Repeat 8 times. Reverse feet and repeat 8 times with right foot forward.

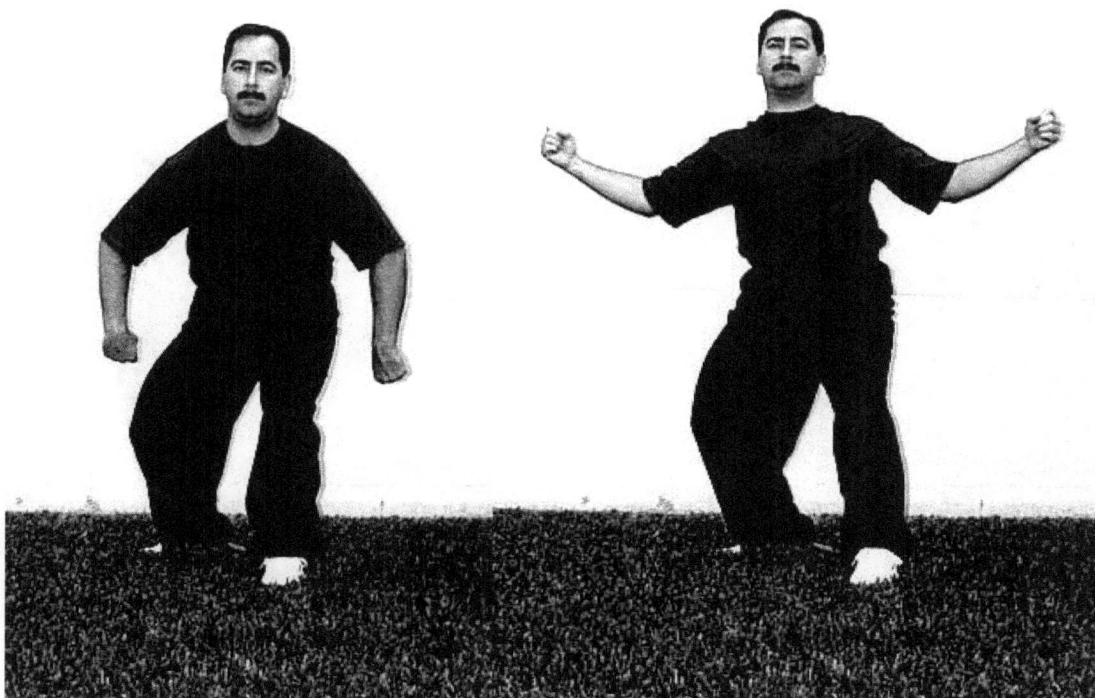

12. **Horizontal Circle - Single Arm** - Left, Right: Left foot forward, right foot back, right hand on hip; **As waist turns**, left arm at chest level elbow not locked extended forward. Hand, palm up with thumb tucked, moves across in front of body from left to right. **Focusing on Tan Tien, movement comes mainly from turning the waist.** Turning palm down, draw hand back in front of head at chin level to beginning point. Repeat 8 times. Reverse feet and repeat with right side 8 times. (Focus: on use of hip motion in a horizontal figure 8)

13. **Horizontal Circles - Doubles**: Optional
(Advanced technique for 2nd year based on Horizontal Circle, Single Arm.)

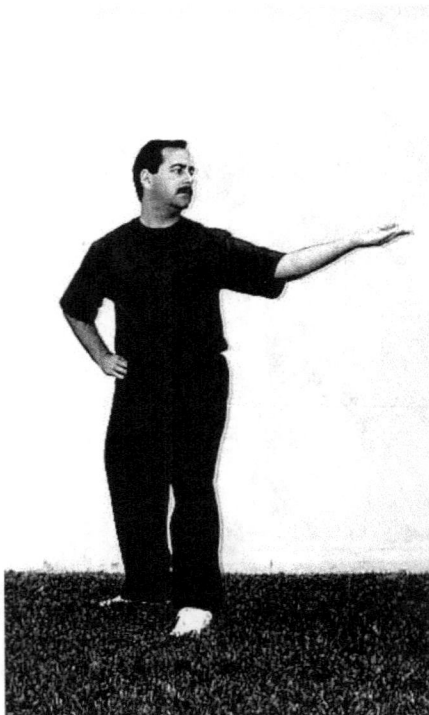

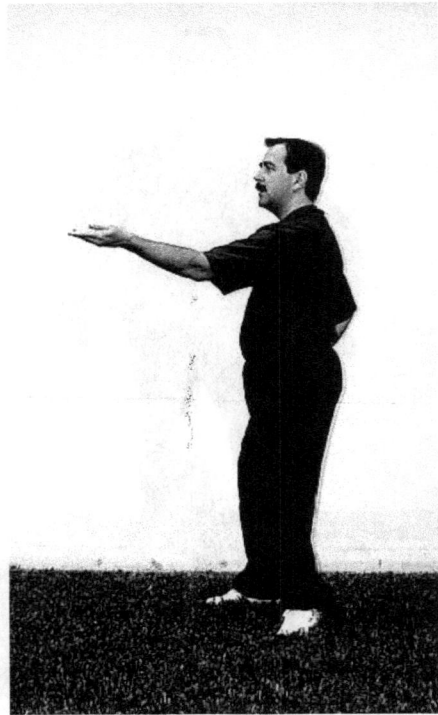

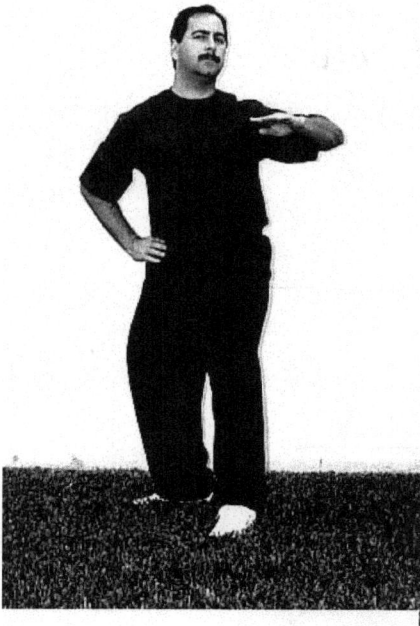
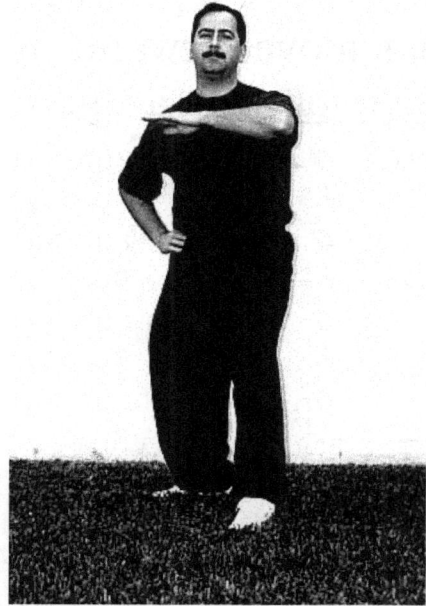
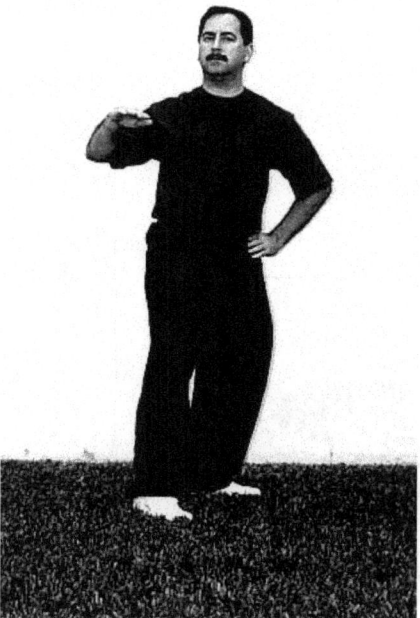
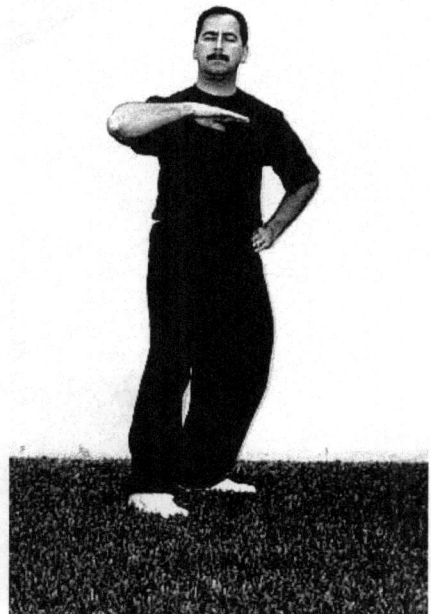

14. **Hips** - Circle Right, Circle Left: Neutral Stance, head up, knees not locked, feet shoulder width apart, hands on hips; Move hips in a horizontal circle, starting from left, hips move forward, right, back and left, 8 times. <u>Reverse direction</u> with a figure 8 and repeat 8 times from right to left.

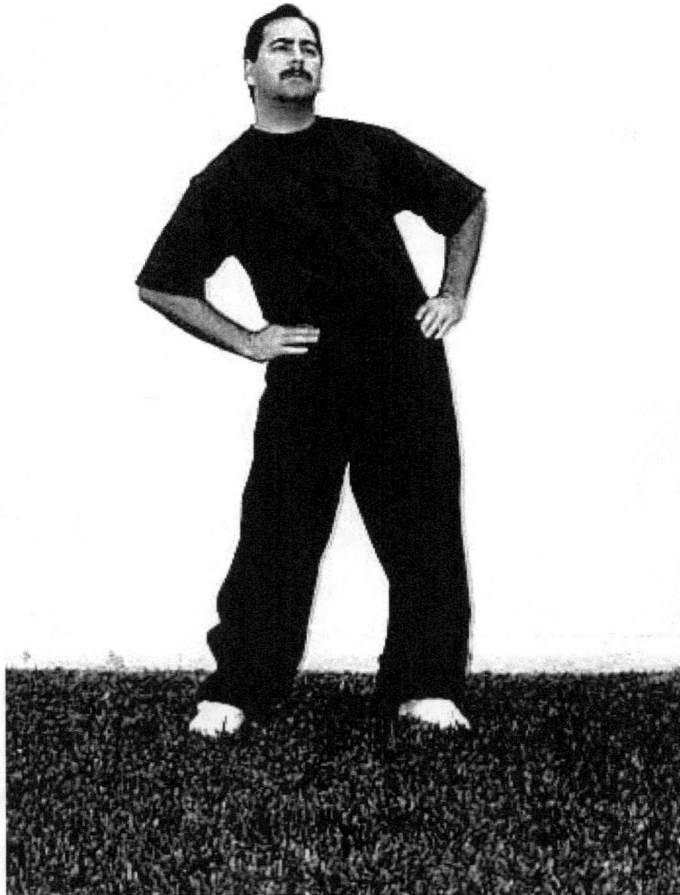

15. **Knees** - Outside/Inside Circles & Forward/Back - Left Side, Right Side: Keeping both feet flat to ground, left foot forward, right foot back, knees not locked, both hands lightly touch left thigh. **As the waist turns from the Tan Tien**, left knee moves right, forward, left and back in a gentle circle. Repeat 8 times in to out. <u>Reverse direction</u> and repeat 8 times out to in with left knee. Straightening left foot, shift weight forward and back. Repeat 8 times. <u>Reverse feet</u> and repeat 8 times in to out and 8 times out to in with the right knee. Straightening right foot, shift weight forward and back. Repeat 8 times.

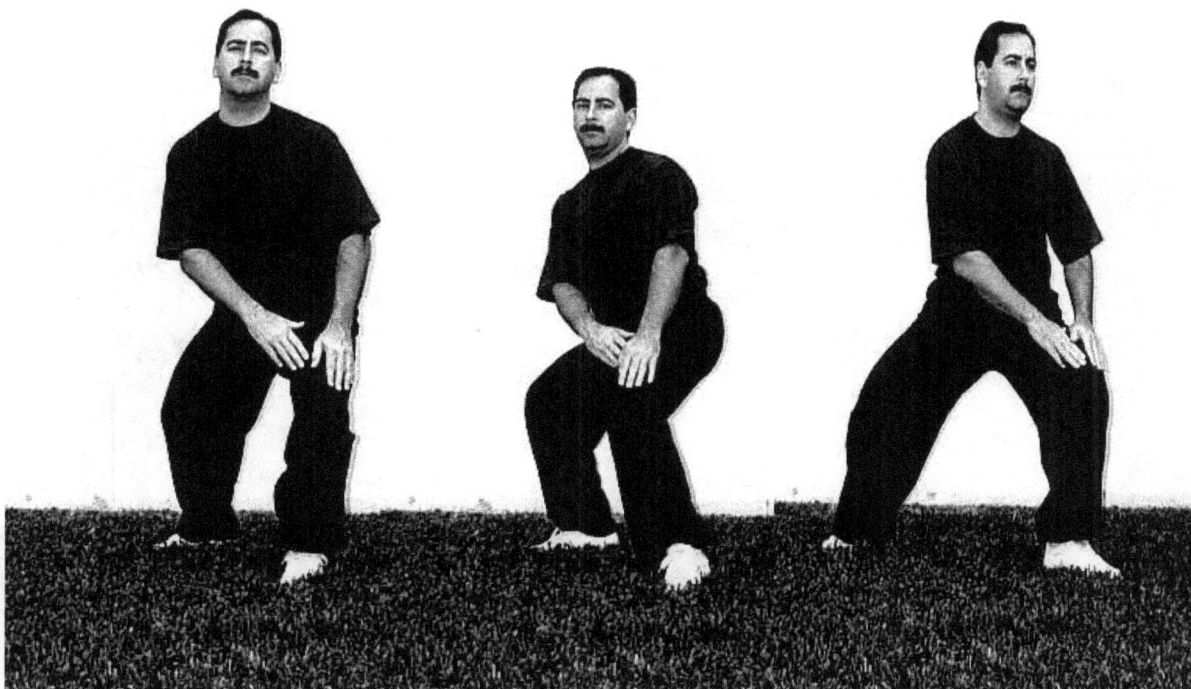

16. **Knees Together** - Circle Right, Circle Left: Hands on top of thighs, fingers lightly touching legs. Move knees in a circle 4 times from left to right; <u>Reverse direction</u>, right to left 4 times.

Knees Apart - Outside, Inside Circles: Repeat with knees apart 4 times in each direction; Knees apart, move knees in to out 4 times; <u>Reverse</u> and move knees out to in 4 times.

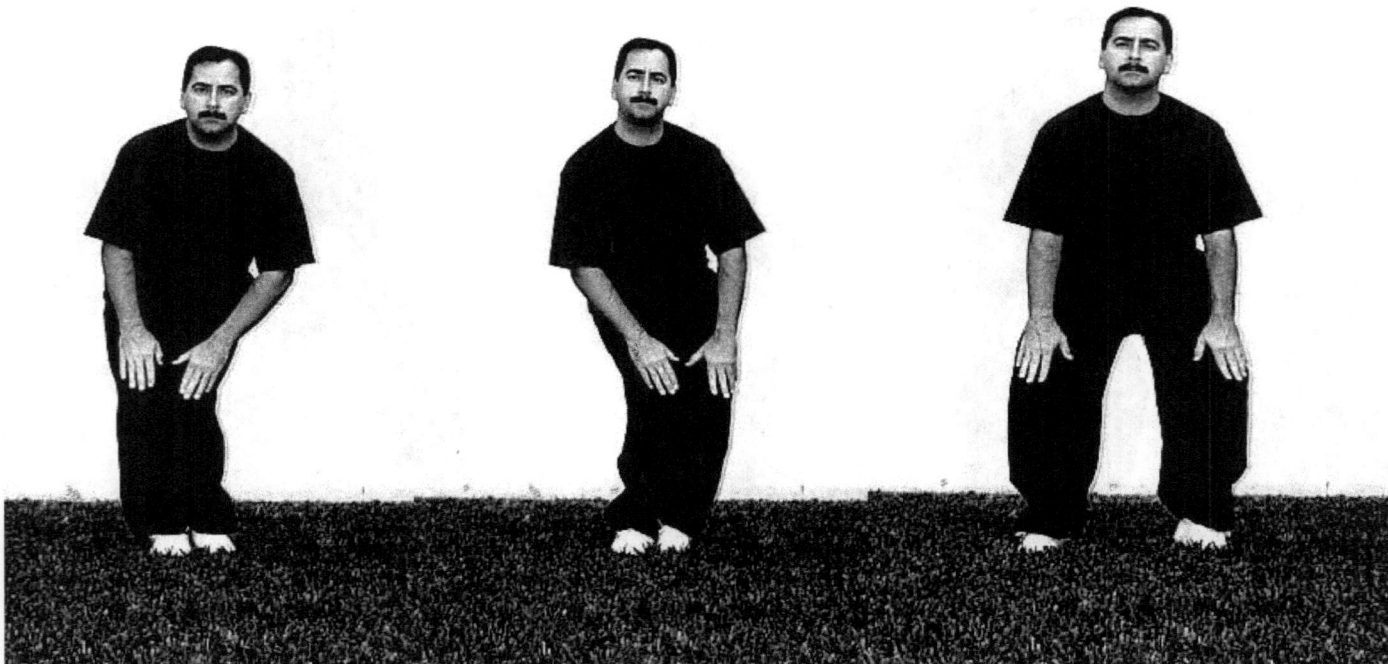

17. **Pick Up Ball**: Neutral Stance, feet shoulder width apart, sink the chi, squat and pick up (imaginary) ball, raise ball in front of body to overhead height. Palms down, lower ball. Palms face one another, finger tips point to sky at uppermost position of exercise. Repeat 8 times beginning with squat. (For strength training, one could use a "medicine" 10# leather ball.)

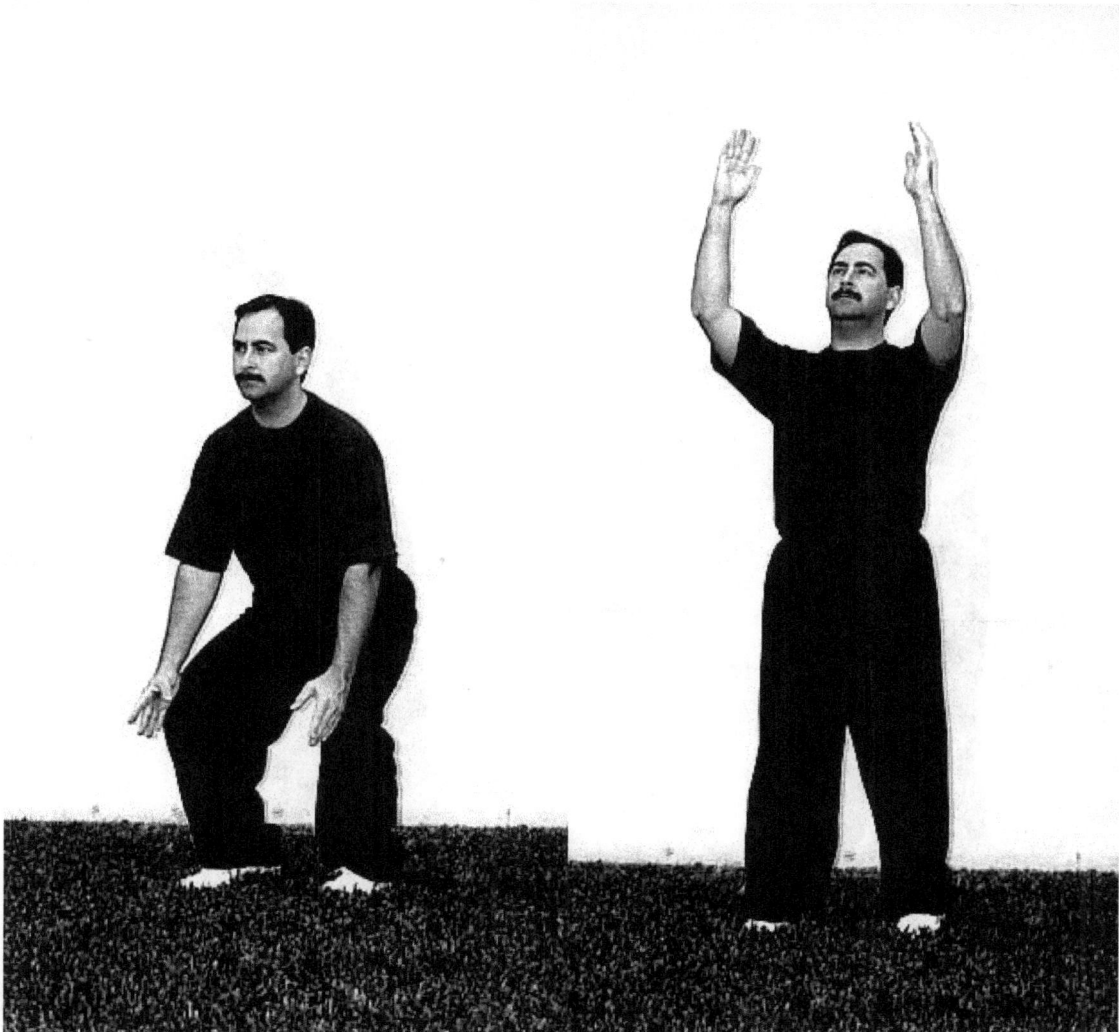

18. **Holding the Ball Circles** - Circle Right, Circle Left: Neutral Stance, feet apart; **As the waist turns**, lift ball over head from left to right in front of body, bring down and across to left to make a circle. Repeat 8 times. <u>Reverse direction</u> with a figure 8 and repeat 8 times. Keep spine aligned; top of head (crown) to sky.

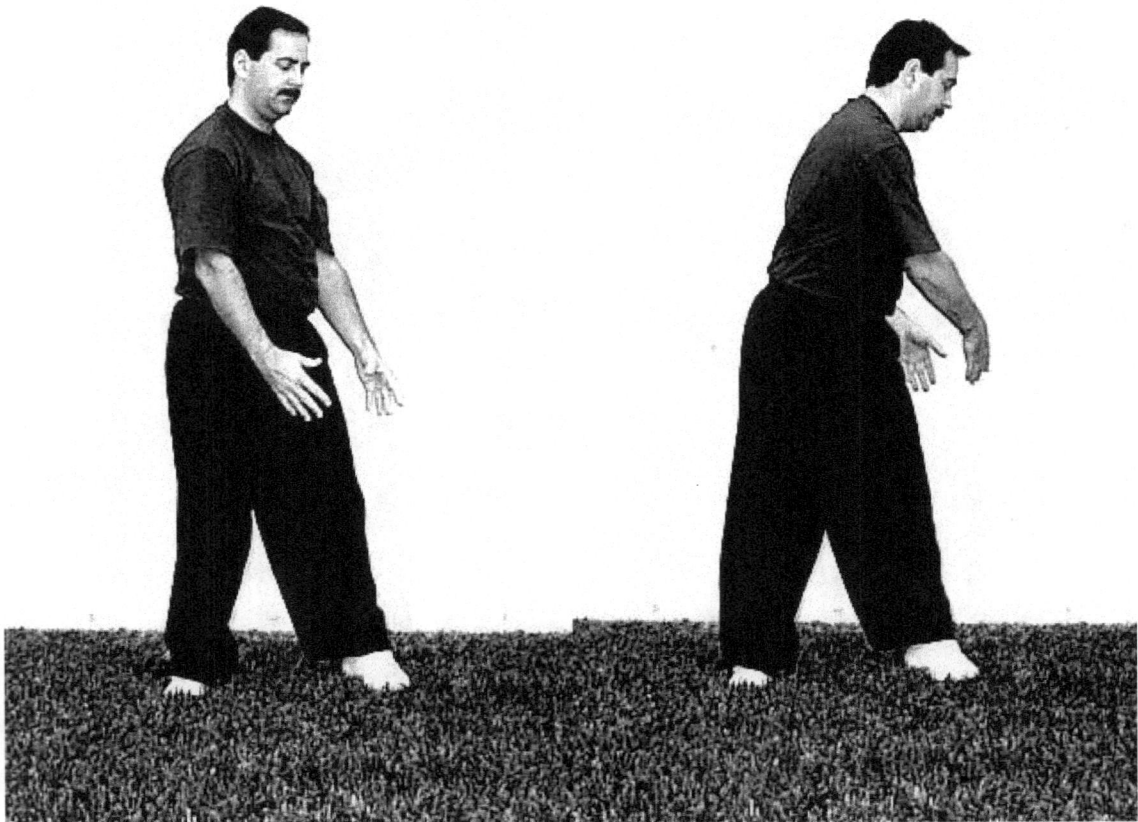

19. **Side Tilt**: Neutral Stance, feet apart, arms extended to sides. Bring left foot in beside right foot; left palm down, right palm up; Bend sideways at waist to the left. As body bends the left hand moves down and behind body, right hand rises to arc above the head. <u>Reversing direction</u>, step to the side with left foot. Bring right foot in beside left foot, left palm up, right palm down; Bend sideways at waist to the right. As the body bends the right hand moves down and behind body, left hand rises to arc above the head. Repeat 8 times.

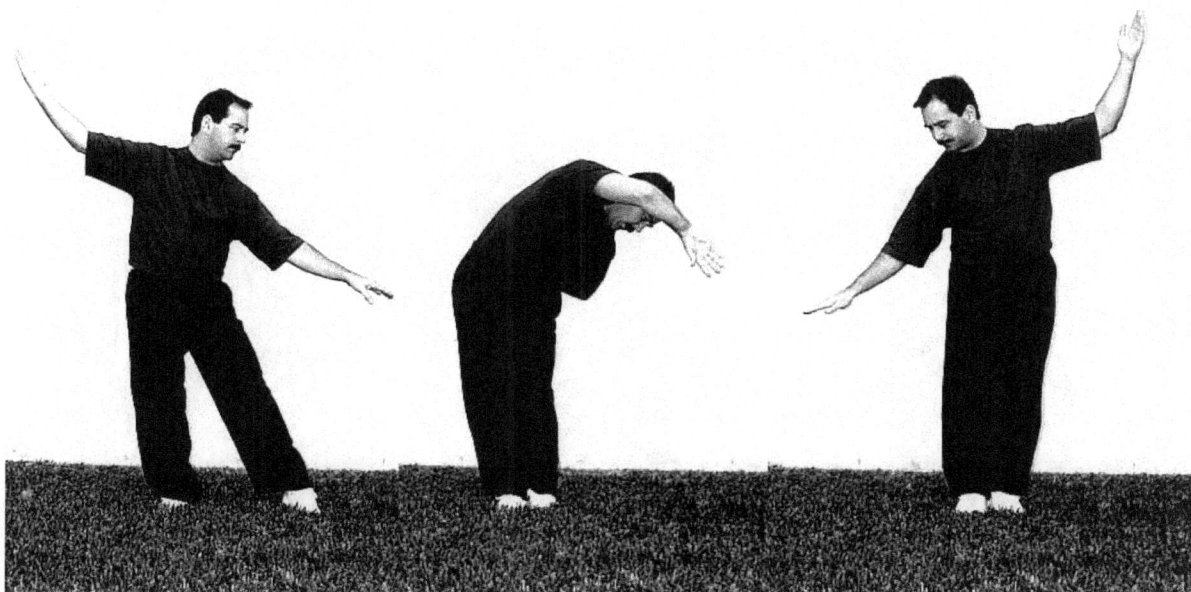

20. **Pat Shoulder**: Neutral Stance, facing front, feet shoulder width apart; arms are extended out at the sides, weight on right foot, lift left toes and pivot on left heel **while turning waist** to left; right foot remains flat, pointing front. Lower left toes keeping heel touching ground. Left knee moves forward slightly but never beyond the point above the toes. Left hand moves down and behind body while right hand moves in front of body and pats left shoulder. Extending arms to sides, lift left toes and pivot on left heel, return to neutral, both feet flat, facing front. Reverse movement to right side.

Alternating Left and Right Sides, repeat for a total of 8 times.

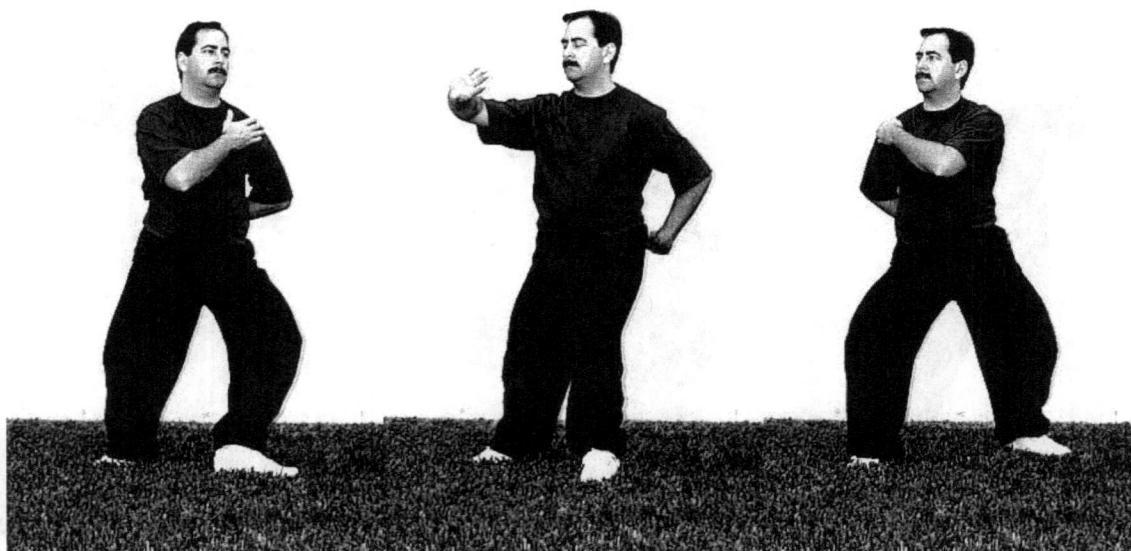

21. **Elbow to Toe**: Neutral Stance, facing front, feet shoulder width apart; As in Pat Shoulder, with weight on right side, lift left toes and pivot on left heel. **As waist turns** to left, arms are folded with right hand inside left elbow. Keeping head up, bend at waist and aim left elbow to upturned left toes. Right foot remains facing front and right knee is bent. Hold for a count of 8. Return to neutral with both feet flat, facing front, arms still folded. Shift weight to left side, fold arms with left hand inside right elbow, lift right toes and pivot to right side. Bend at waist and aim right elbow to upturned right toes. Hold for a count of 8.

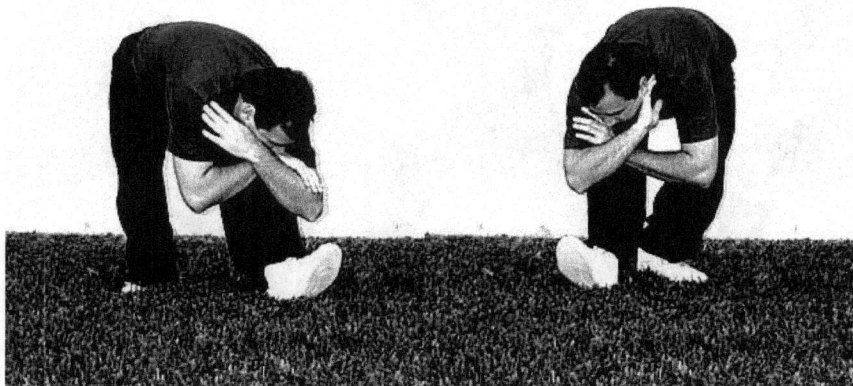

22. **Polish the Mirror**: In a Horse Stance, hands move towards each other, fingertips leading, palms up, until fingers almost touch and backs of hands are together with knuckles nearly touching. Hands rise in front of body, parting near top of head. Palms press forward, away from body, hands turning down, arms extend to each side as arms lower and come together again in front of the body. Left arm moves in a counter clockwise circle and right arm in clockwise circle. Repeat 4 times.

Reverse direction. Hands, back to back, lower in front of body. Hands part at bottom of circle, arms extended to sides, palms turn up. Hands rise in wide circle to come together at top of circle. Repeat 4 times.

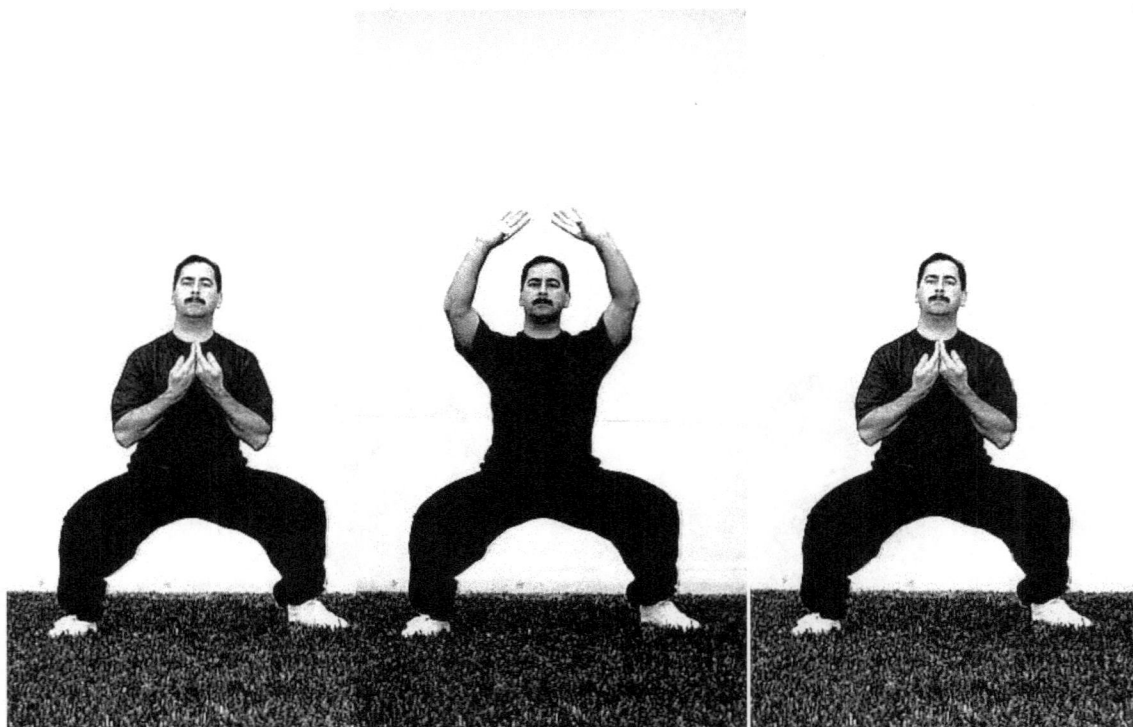

23. **Grind Corn**: In a Horse Stance, circle hands horizontally to right, then left. Palms down, right hand slightly above left hand. As the waist turns, hands move to right, left hand rises and right hand lowers. As waist turns, hands move to left. <u>Reverse direction</u> and as waist turns, complete circle is repeated. Leading hand is always above following hand.

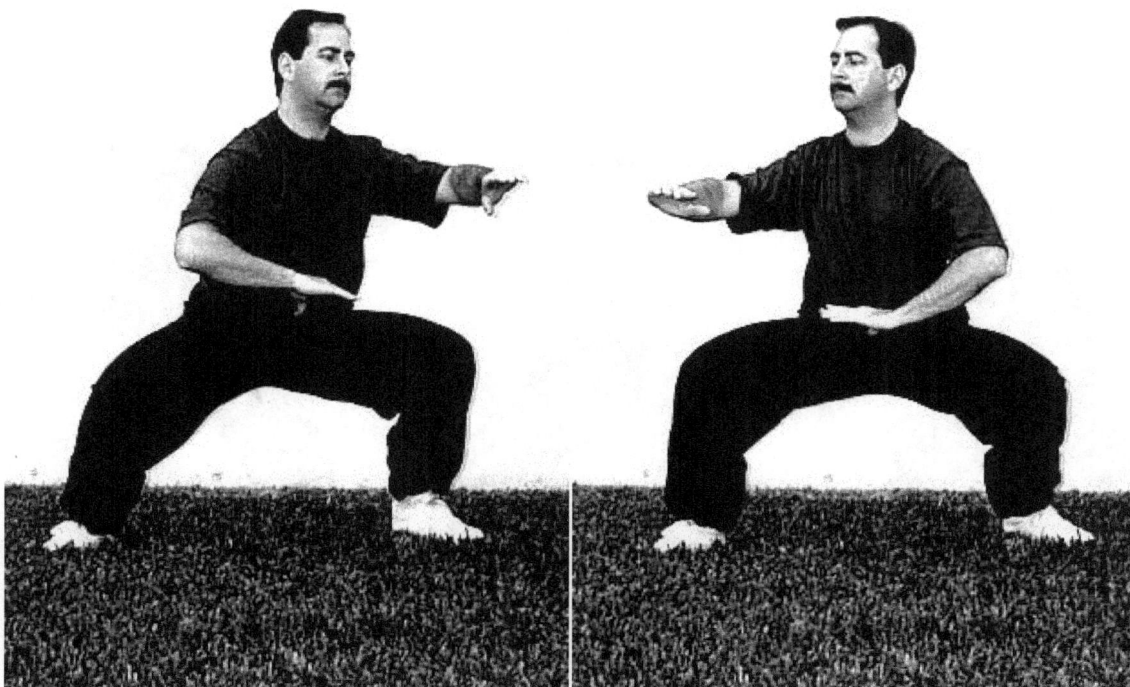

24. **Look Over Shoulder** - Left Side, Right Side: In a Horse Stance, fingertips point toward one another without touching, in front of body with palms down. As waist turns, hands rise on left to a point above head with fingertips almost touching creating a vertical circle in front of the body. At top of circle palms are up. Hands lower and cross in front of body. Parting, left hand goes behind back, palm out; while right hand presses away from left shoulder. Turn waist, look over left shoulder.

<u>Reverse direction</u> of circle by turning from waist, circling motion ends with right hand behind back and left hand presses away from right shoulder.

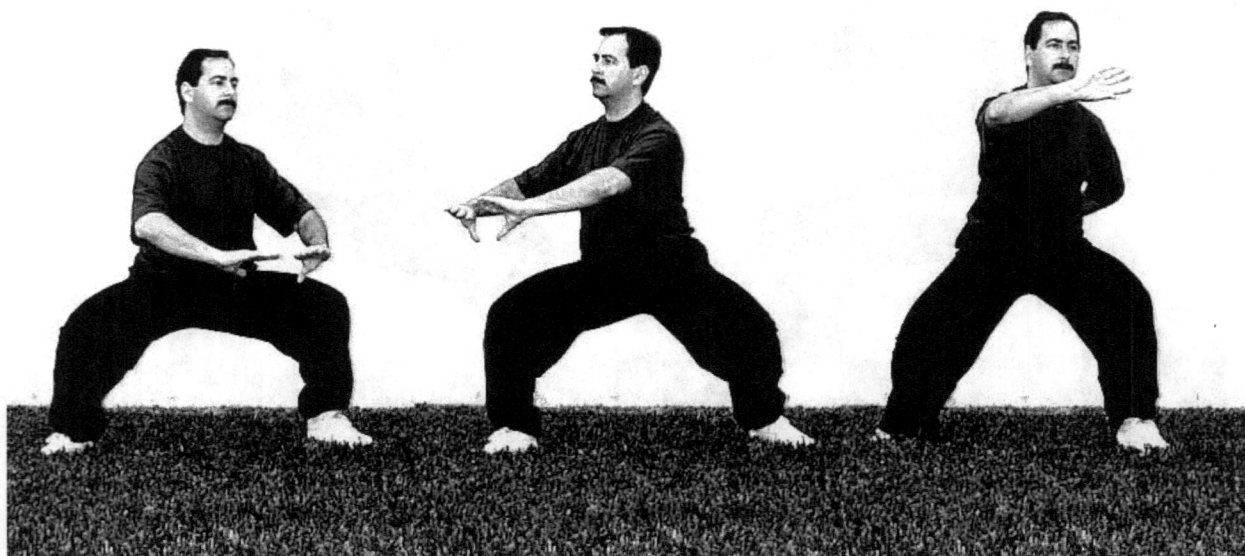

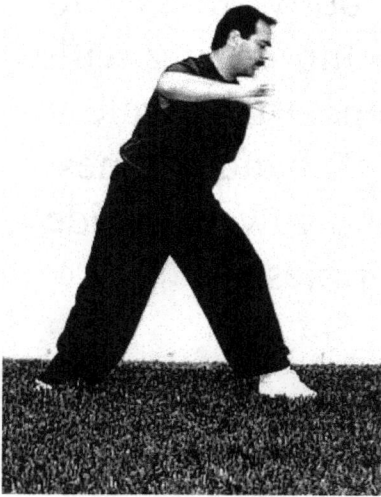

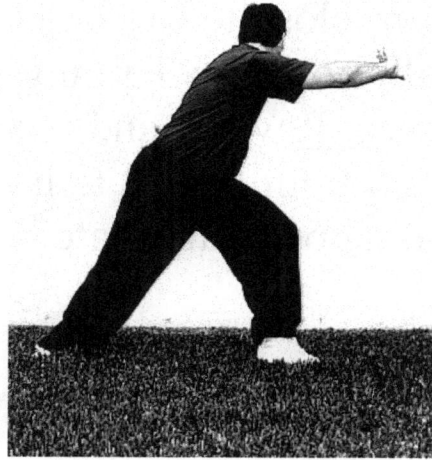

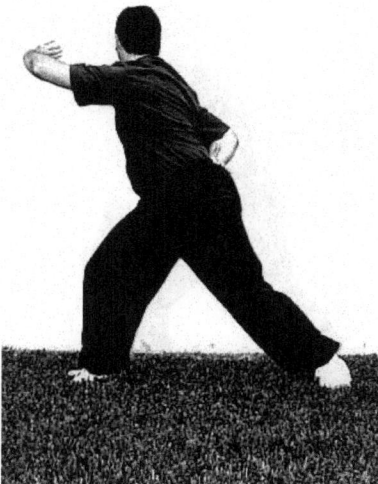

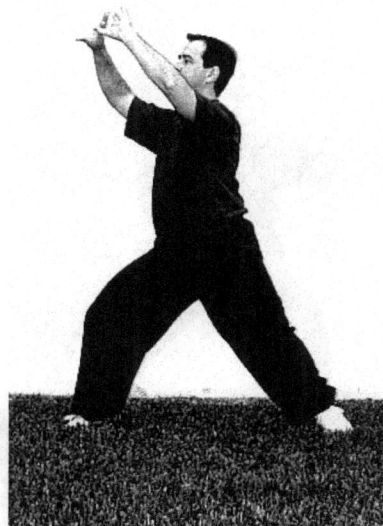

25. **Snake Arm** - Right Side, Left Side, Alternating Together: In a Horse Stance, with left hand on hip, right hand rises palm up, arm extended to side. Hand, palm down, thumb tucked when beside the body, moves to skim close to the body from shoulder to hip ending with palm to back. Turning palms back up repeat the circle 8 times. <u>Reverse</u> and repeat motion with left hand 8 times. With both hands, rising side palm up, and lowering side palm down, alternate hands and repeat 8 times.

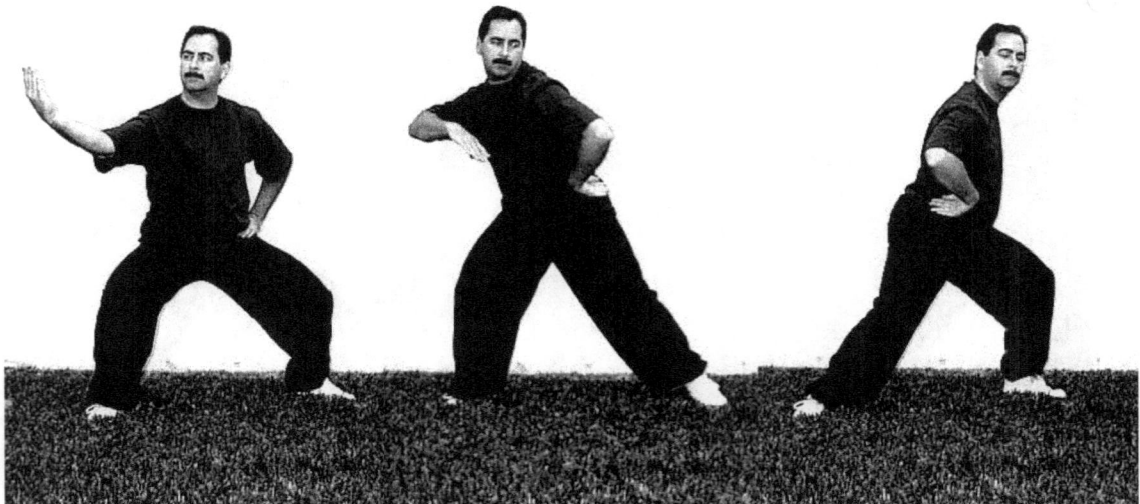

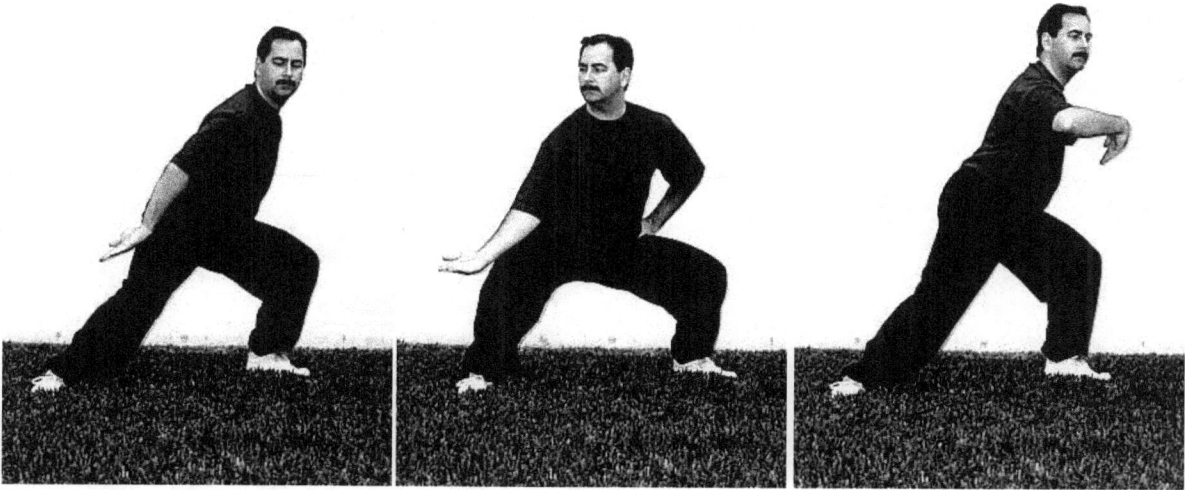

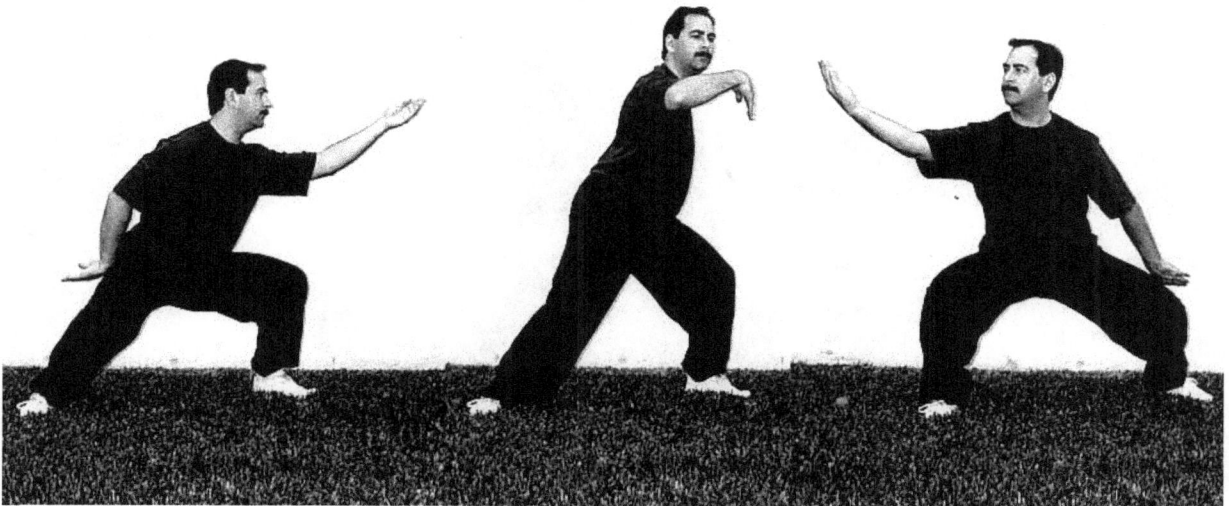

26. **Shake the Chi**: In a Neutral Stance, feet apart, firmly rooted. Cleanse, Catch the Chi in front of body.Shake loosely closed fists with arms in embrace position. Waist and shoulders all move. (variation: roll forearms from embrace position, knuckles aligning in front of body.)

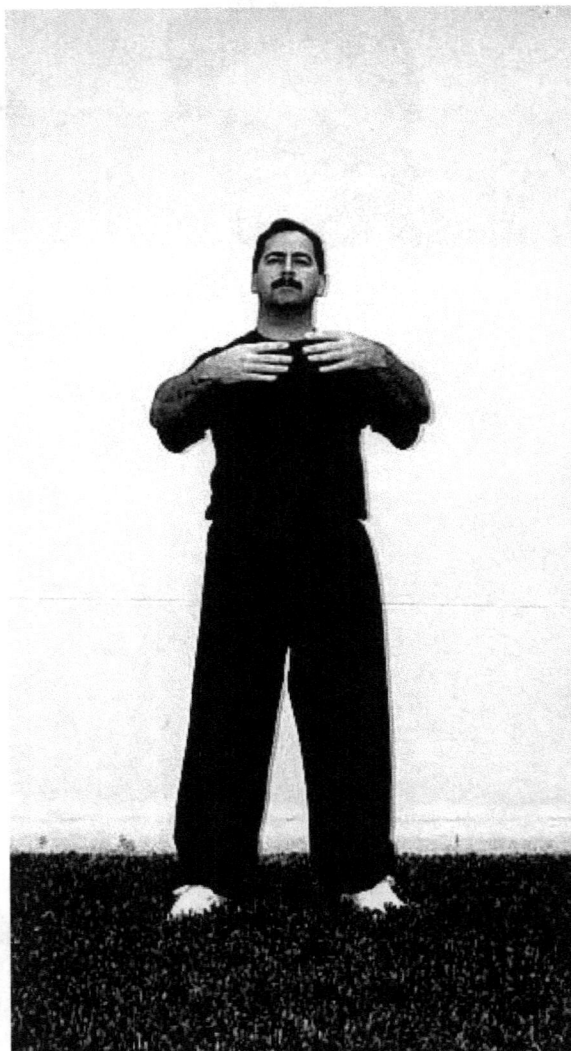

27. **Standing Meditation** - Three Hand Postures: Neutral Stance, knees slightly bent or relaxed, feet apart. Eyes are closed during this exercise if comfortable. Hands extended in front of hips, palms down (Earth). Hold posture for count of 8*; Slowly turn palms up (Sky). Hold for count of 8. Lifting elbows, point fingers toward each other, almost but not quite touching; arms are rounded as though in an embrace (Human). Maintain roundness of circle, relax shoulders. Hold for count of 8. Cleanse.

*Advanced work: postures are held for any amount of time up to 1 hour.

Closing: Shift weight right, slight bend of right knee. Bring left leg beside right leg. Bow to close.

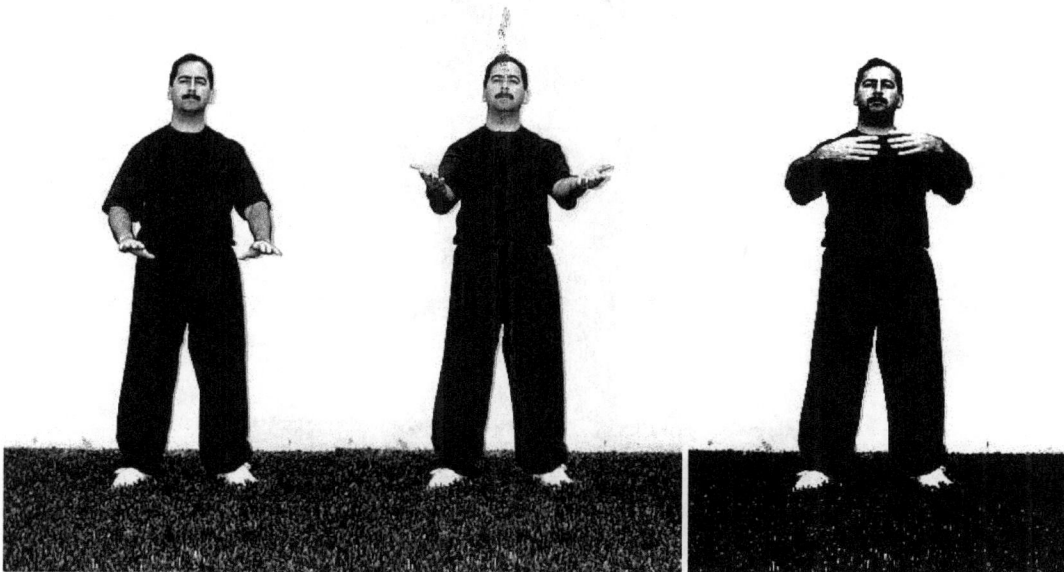

28. **Wu Chi**: Heels together, knees slightly bent or relaxed "not locked", feet, toes slightly apart. Eyes are closed (if able or comfortable). Meditate by focusing mentally to lower Tan Tien. Focus on breathing from Tan Tien. Relax, yet maintain posture. Hold for count of 8. (Advanced work: Hold posture for any amount of time or up to 1 hour.)

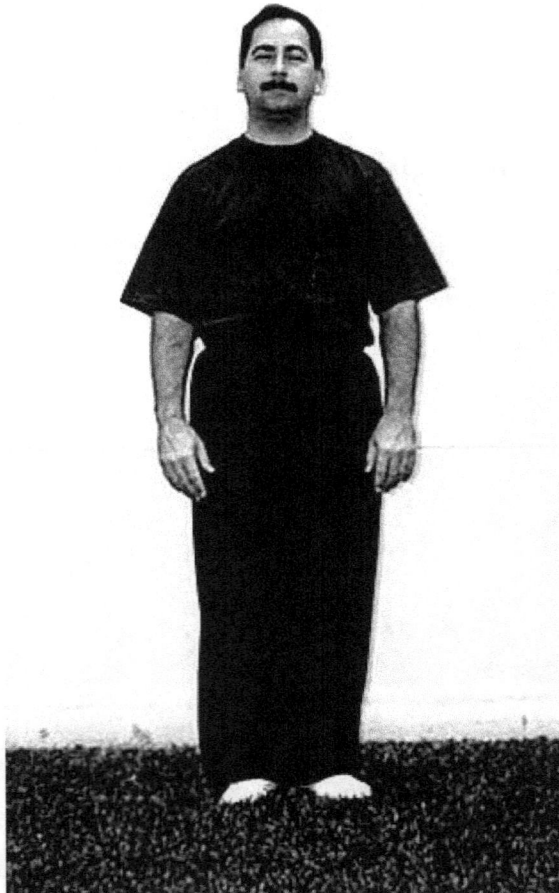

Stances

Horse Stance: Arms embracing form a large round circle in front of body; fingertips point to one another without touching: To assume horse stance, start with heels together forming a 'V' or 45 degree angle, facing front. Alternately move first heels, then toes out in a zigzag pattern five times, ending with heels. Feet are spread apart approximately twice one's shoulder width. Press heels slightly out, then lower the body as though sitting in a saddle. In the beginning, do not try to go any lower than is comfortable.

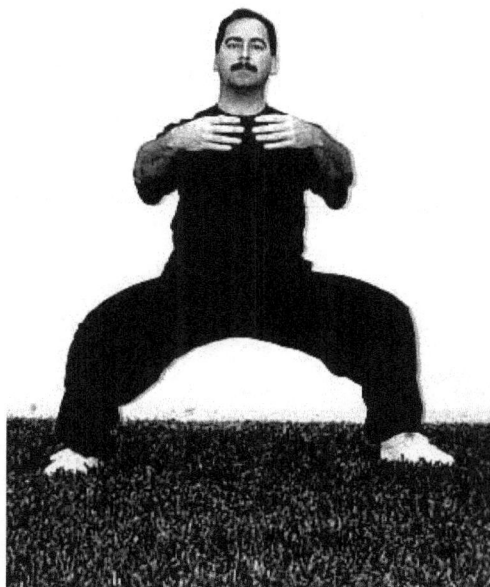

Bow Stance - Right Side Forward, Left Side Forward: Begin in Horse Stance, shift weight right, move left toes toward center, pivot on left heel. Place weight on left foot, turn waist, lift right toes, pivot on right heel, adjust right foot by rooting from left foot. (Advanced students, weight should be 60% on the right leg. Knee should be bent so "ideally" the right thigh is parallel to the ground.) Right foot is toed in. The right knee does not go past the toes.

The right palm extends away from the body, fingers point to the sky. Head is turned toward right hand. Eyes look over the fingers lined up in a row. Extend the thumb and the index finger to create the "Tiger's Mouth". (Optional, the eyes may look between the thumb and index finger, through the "Tiger's Mouth".) The left hand is drawn back as if on a bow. Extend fingers of left hand pointing to the earth, the thumb tucks at the Tan Tien or belt region. This completes Right Side Forward.

<u>Left Side Forward</u>: Using the same principles described, change to other side. Reverse the placement of the feet and hands.

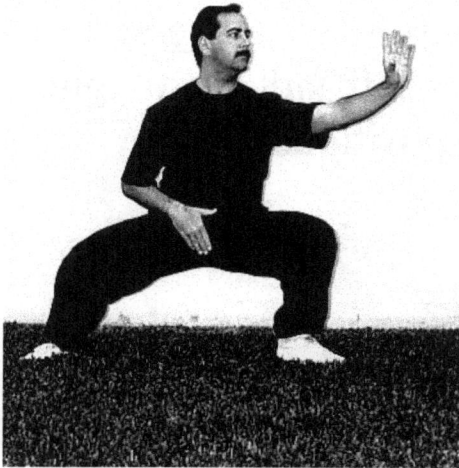 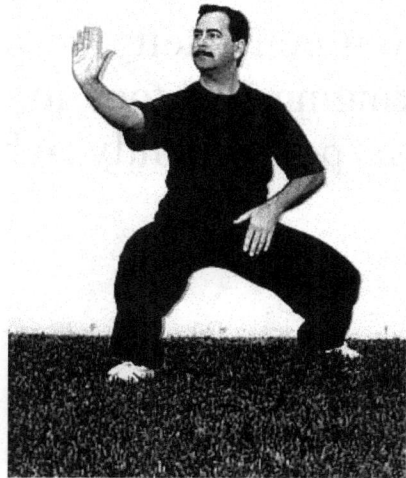

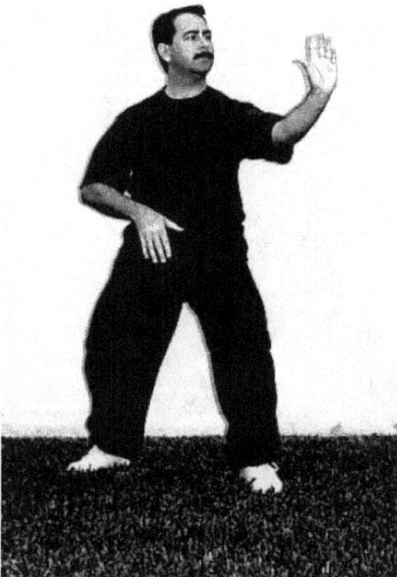 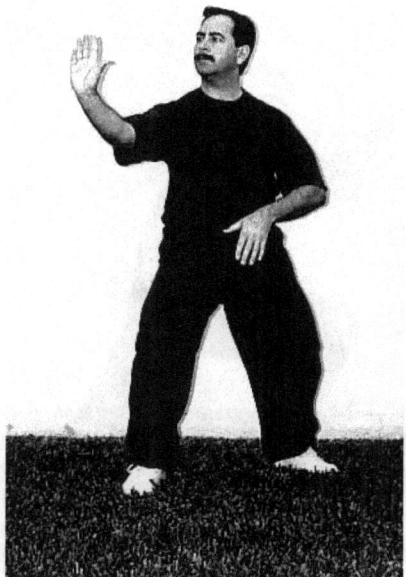

Back Stance - Left and Right Side: Feet shoulder width apart; feet flat to ground (can also be in lower posture or horse stance); knees bent; Weight on right side; Left toes point slightly left, right toes point forward; Right fist up, palm out, even with eyebrow, arms rounded, press away from body; left fist, palm down at hip level. <u>Reverse</u> by bringing left toes in, shift weight to left side and right toes point slightly right. Reverse fist positions.

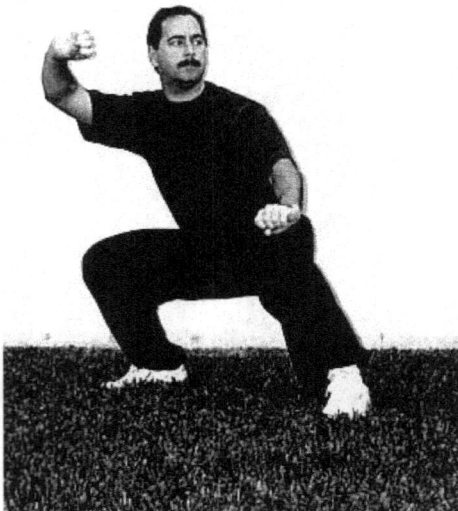

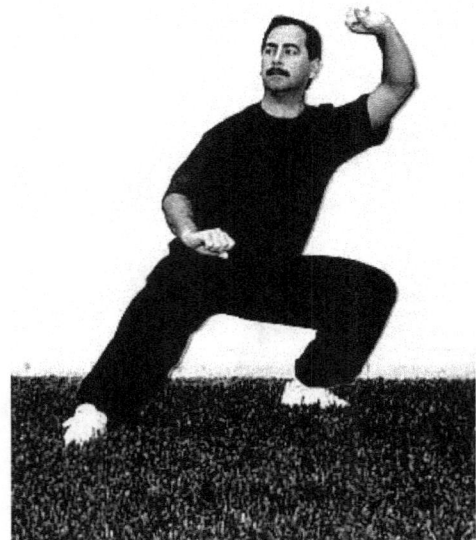

7-Star Stance (Play Guitar) - Left and Right Side: Left foot forward with toes raised, heel touching ground, right foot back, flat on ground, toes pointing to right, weight on right side, slight natural bend in knees. Arms extended to front with natural bend at elbows, palms in. Left hand forward, right hand slightly lower and back. <u>Reverse</u>: weight on left; right foot forward, toes up, heel touching ground, left foot back, flat, toes point left. Right hand forward, left hand slightly lower and back.

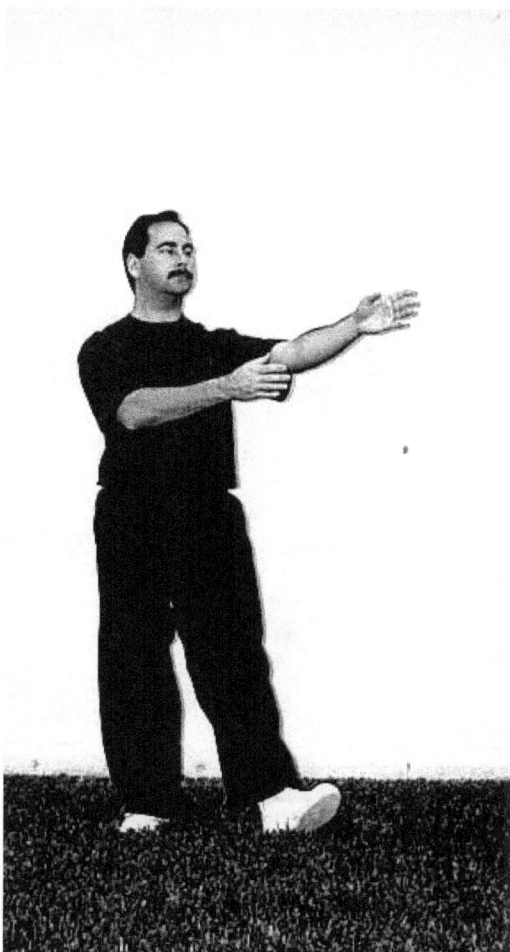

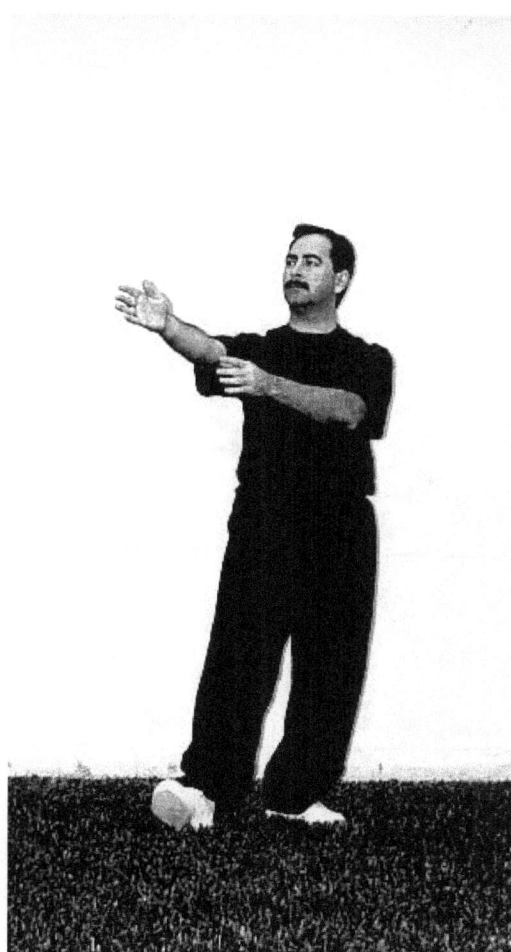

Cat Stance - Left and Right Side: Weight on right side; right foot flat, pointing slightly right; knees slightly bent. Left foot forward with only toes or ball of foot touching ground. Rounding the arms, left hand back, fingers touching to form a point, (Crane's Beak) hooks behind back. Right hand, palm out, pressing forward and away from right eyebrow. <u>Change Posture</u> by placing left foot flat in Neutral Stance, shift weight to left side. Extend right foot forward, toes touch ground, right hand, in Crane's Beak, hooks behind back. Left hand, palm out, pressing forward and away from left eyebrow.

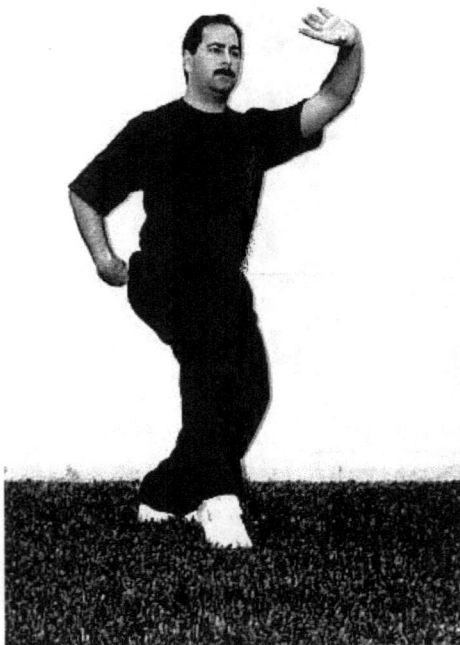

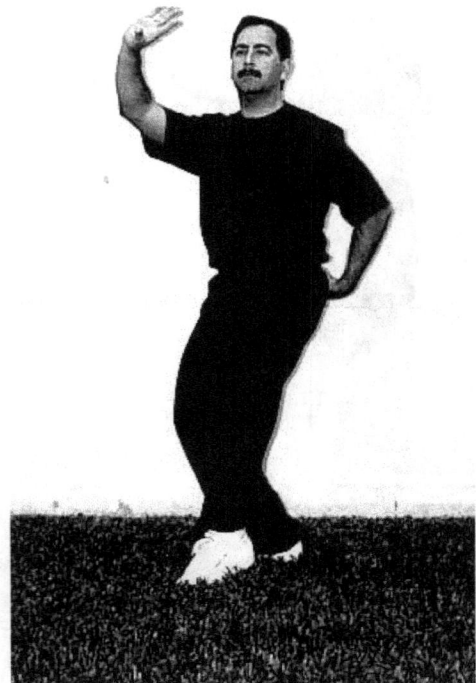

Single Leg Stance - Left and Right Side: Weight on right side; right foot flat, pointing to right side; Left foot forward with toes touching; Right fist pressing away from ear, extended above eyebrow; Left fist, palm down at hip level above left thigh; Slowly lift left knee and hold posture. Lower left foot and shift weight to left side. Reverse foot and hand positions; slowly lift right knee and hold. If it is not possible to lift leg, hold stance using the cat footwork instead.

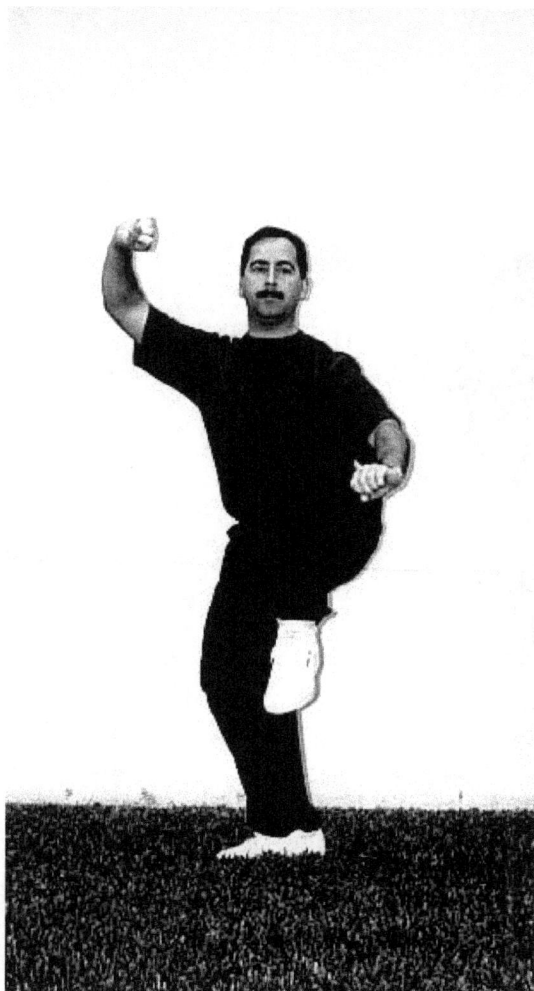

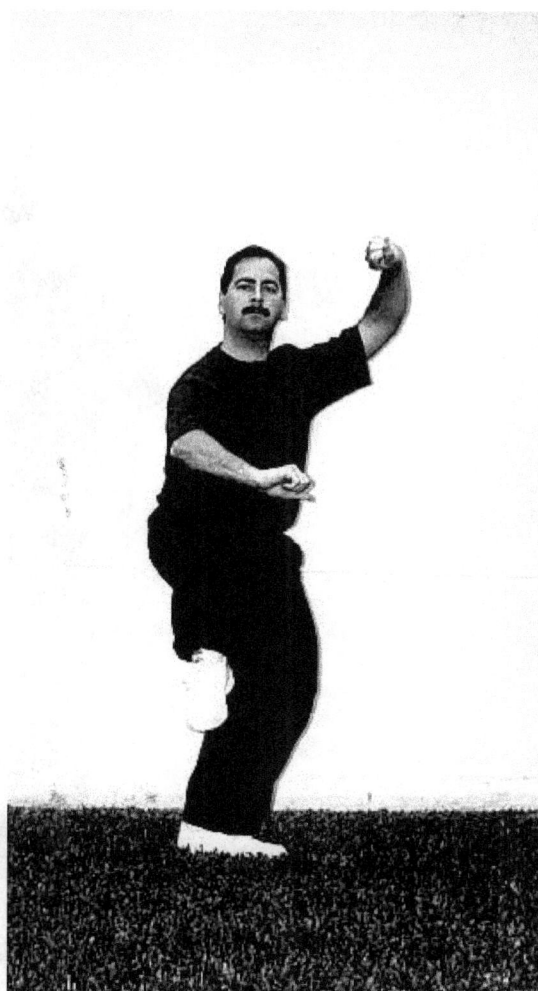

Wu Chi: Heels together, feet slightly apart forming a 'V' shape, face and eyes looking forward, arms relaxed at sides. Close eyes if comfortable, mentally focus on lower Tan Tien; breathing is full, relaxed and natural, originating from Tan Tien.

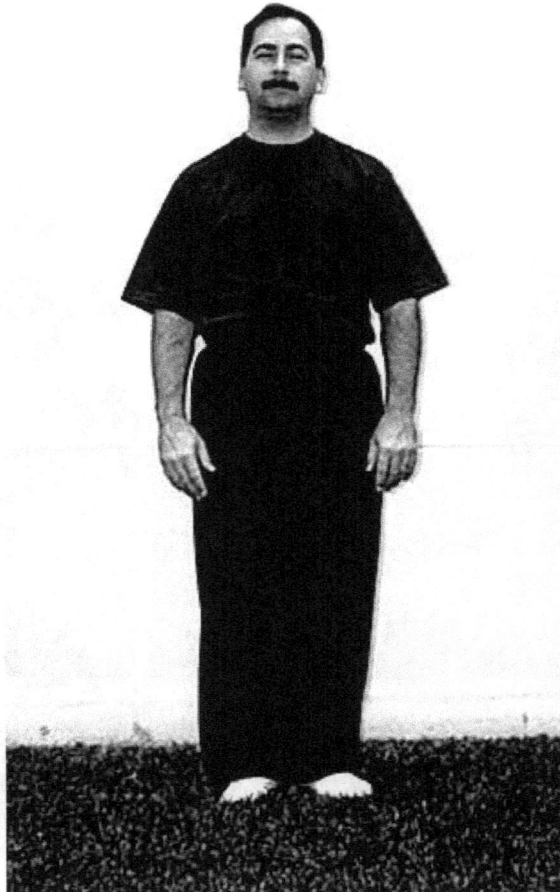

Glossary

Chan Ssi Ching or **Tzan Tzi Chin** - English translation: "Silk Reeling Spiraling Power Exercises".

Chen Style Tai Chi Chuan - The Chen family is considered the origin of formalized traditional Tai Chi Chuan.

Chi - Vital life energy.

Circle - Everything in Nature has a circle aspect.

Cleansing - To be made clean or fresh; to rid oneself of negative or stagnant energy (chi).

Crane's Beak - The fingertips of one hand touching to form a point. Resembles a Cranes Beak. The wrist and elbow remain slightly bent (not locked).

Dragon - A style of Chinese martial arts based upon the movements of the dragon.

Kung Fu - "Effort and Time". Skill or achievement acquired over time.

Meditation - State of relaxation.

Pa Kua Chang (Ba Gua) - "Eight Changing Palms". An internal martial art style based upon the Tai Chi Circle.

Sifu - Teacher.

Silk Reeling - Reference made to the smoothness needed to unravel a cocoon of the silk worm.

Snake - A style of Chinese kung fu based upon the movements of the snake; using twisting, coiling and spiraling movements; rhythmic undulations.

Spiral - Curving, coiling, circling twisting and twining movements based upon the concept of the Yin/Yang or Tai Chi Circle.

Stance (Posture) - A position in which the body is held or maintained with good alignment of the human structure.

Tai Chi Chuan - Ancient Chinese meditative movements practiced as a system of exercises.

Tan Tien - (pronounced don tee-en) Literal translation means "Field of Elixir" or "Energy Field". A spherical area in the body capable of storing and generating chi. The (Lower) Tan Tien is located a few inches below the navel.

Taoist - One who practices being in Harmony with the Universe and all Nature.

Wu Chi - A state of "Unattached Awareness".

Index

About the Author's Teacher

Master Frank J. Paolillo is a certified teacher (Sifu) of the Shantung Arts of China. He has studied with several of China's finest teachers including the world famous Martial Arts Grandmaster Poi Chan of Sha Cheng; Internal Arts Master Kay Chi Leung, Doctor of Acupuncture, Taiwan; Master Li En Jiu of Jinan, Tai Chi Grandchampion and coach of China's National Team; Tai Chi and Chi Kung Master Zhang Xue Xin of Beijing; and Pa Kua expert Hing Lun Kwan of Zhengzhou.

Sifu Paolillo's instruction includes the cultivation of chi (inner energy) through Taoist Meditation and Chi Kung, the silk-like spiraling movements of Chen Tai Chi Chuan and the twisting and circling movements of Dragon Pa Kua Chang. He teaches Northern Praying Mantis Kung Fu and Shantung weapons training to further enhance awareness, agility, centering and manifestation of energy to power.

His focus is on meditative movement and internal martial arts for the self-awareness of human nature and the integration of body/mind/spirit. His methods of training are based on "returning to nature" techniques derived from the internal arts of China.

About the Author

Paul Ellsworth was born at Ft. Bragg, North Carolina, January 23, 1963, in the year of the Water Tiger. His father was in the U.S. Air Force (retired Major). His family also lived in Hawaii and Oklahoma during his father's military active duty. Paul has a Bachelor of Arts degree in Religion with minors in Biological and Chemical Sciences from Florida State University (1986). While attending FSU, Paul was a member of the World Renowned Marching Chiefs. He played trumpet. He is a member of Alpha Chi Sigma (AXE), a professional chemistry fraternity. He has completed courses in Life Insurance, Health Insurance, Variable Annuities, Mutual Fund Sales (NASD Series 6) and Real Estate. He has taken graduate courses in Business Law, Intergovernmental Relations, Capitalism and Human Values, Science, Technology and Society.

Paul began his formal training in Martial Arts in 1991 from Master F.J. Paolillo. In addition to Silk Reeling, he has studied Chen style Tai Chi Chuan, Northern Praying Mantis, Snake, Dragon style Pa Kua Chang (Ba Gua), various Shantung weapons such as: double-edged sword, broadsword, staff, spear, cane, kwan do, and other internal Taoist arts. Paul received permission from his "Sifu" to teach and has taught numerous Tai Chi and Chi Kung classes since 1995. He currently lives near the Atlantic Ocean in Florida.

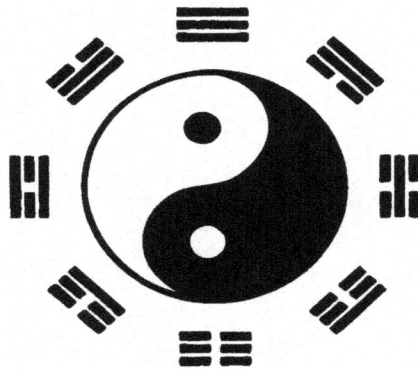

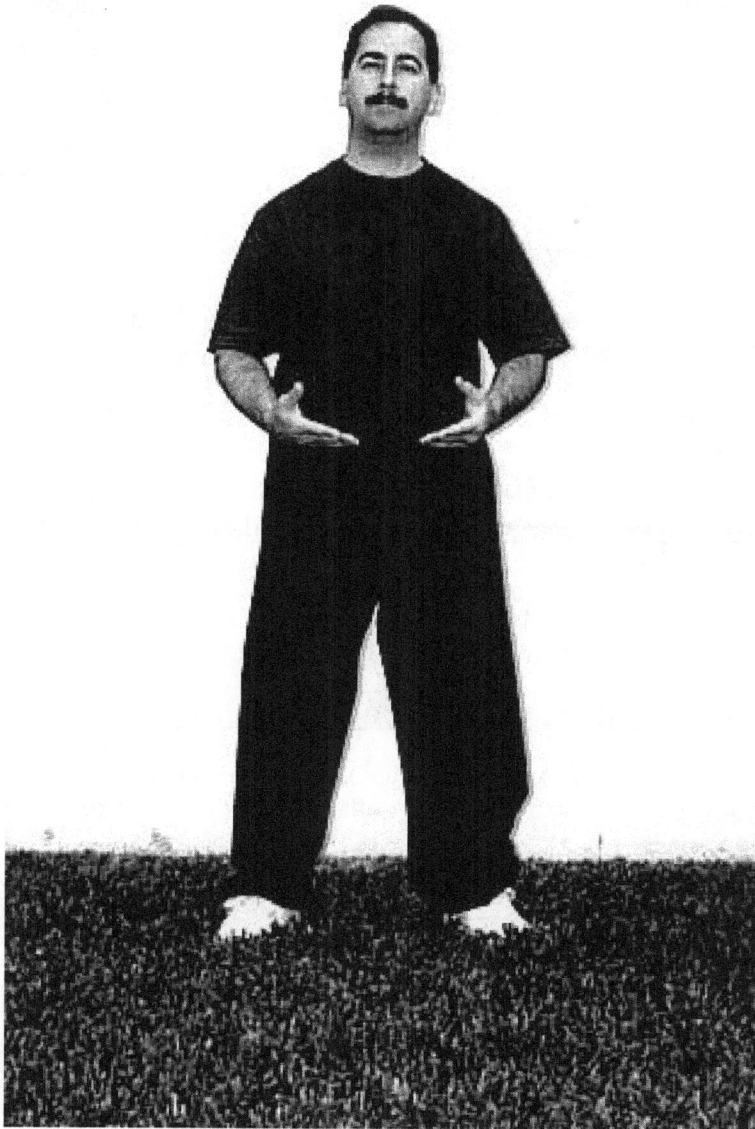

Order Form

To order **Tai Chi Chuan Silk Reeling Exercises** directly from the publisher, fill out this form, enclose a check or money order and mail to:

Jade Emperor Publishing
P.O. Box 51541
Jacksonville Beach, Florida 32240-1541, USA

Please send _____ copy(ies) of **Tai Chi Chuan Silk Reeling Exercises** @ $19.95 Plus $6.00 shipping per copy to:

This book may be returned in an undamaged, like new, resalable condition to this publisher for a full refund if returned within 3 days after receiving with cash register receipt/shipping invoice.

SHIP TO: Name:_____   Price per copy: _____

Address:_____   Sales Tax and S & H:_____

City/State/Zip _____   Total Enclosed:_____
Telephone:_____

ORDERS SHIPPED VIA PRIORITY MAIL.

SALES TAX: Add 7.0% sales tax per book for orders shipped to Florida addresses.
PAYMENT: We accept checks or money orders. Make payable to Jade Emperor Publishing. Include sales tax, if applicable. (Prices Subject to Change without Notice)
IF THIS IS A LIBRARY BOOK, PLEASE PHOTOCOPY THIS ORDER FORM.

....

Order Form

To order **Tai Chi Chuan Silk Reeling Exercises** directly from the publisher, fill out this form, enclose a check or money order and mail to:

Jade Emperor Publishing
P.O. Box 51541
Jacksonville Beach, Florida 32240-1541, USA

Please send _____ copy(ies) of **Tai Chi Chuan Silk Reeling Exercises** @ $19.95 Plus $6.00 shipping per copy to:

This book may be returned in an undamaged, like new, resalable condition to this publisher for a full refund if returned within 3 days after receiving with cash register receipt/shipping invoice.

SHIP TO: Name:_____   Price per copy: _____

Address:_____   Sales Tax and S & H:_____

City/State/Zip _____   Total Enclosed:_____
Telephone:_____

ORDERS SHIPPED VIA PRIORITY MAIL.

SALES TAX: Add 7.0% sales tax per book for orders shipped to Florida addresses.
PAYMENT: We accept checks or money orders. Make payable to Jade Emperor Publishing. Include sales tax, if applicable. (Prices Subject to Change without Notice)
IF THIS IS A LIBRARY BOOK, PLEASE PHOTOCOPY THIS ORDER FORM.

....

www.ingramcontent.com/pod-product-compliance
Lightning Source LLC
Chambersburg PA
CBHW081724270326
41933CB00017B/3289